Peter Moy • Patrick Palacci • Ingvar Ericsson

Immediate Function & Esthetics in Implant Dentistry

Immediate Function & Esthetics in Implant Dentistry

Edited by
Peter Moy
Patrick Palacci
Ingvar Ericsson

Quintessence Publishing Co. Ltd.
London, Berlin, Chicago, Tokyo, Barcelona, Istanbul, Milan, Moscow,
New-Delhi, Paris, Beijing, Prague, São Paulo, Seoul, and Warsaw

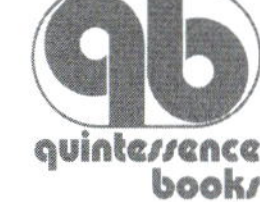

Quintessence

British Library Cataloguing in Publication Data

Moy, Peter K.
Immediate function esthetics in implant dentistry
1. Dental implants
I. Title II. Palacci, Patrick III. Ericcson, Ingvar
617.6'93

ISBN-13: 9781850971733

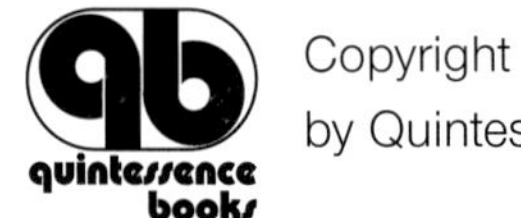

Printing and Binding: fgb freiburger graphische betriebe
ISBN: 978-1-85097-173-3
Printed in Germany

Foreword

General technical developments, especially in the area of computers, have led to new and fascinating tools becoming available for medicine and dentistry.

Contemporary methods within radiology, such as computerized tomography and medical imaging, have made patient information available for diagnosis in a totally new way. Furthermore, ongoing development has made these technologies less costly and therefore more readily available for doctors and patients.

Guided surgery is an example of a technology that has developed in this way. The utilization of new powerful technologies has to be conducted in close consultation with experienced clinicians. The technology is just a tool, no matter how powerful.

This book describes and documents how to use NobelGuide™ in various clinical situations. It is based on long-term clinical ambitions, thorough knowledge of the development of this technology, and the ambition to strive for what is the best for the patient.

Matts Andersson, DDS PhD
Chief Scientist, Nobel Biocare AB
Gothenburg

Preface

Professor Per Ingvar Brånemark first introduced the concept and principles of osseointegration to North America during the Toronto Conference in 1982 after years of research and clinical trials. The protocol presented at that time recommended a non-loaded healing period of between 3 and 6 months for dental implants. These recommendations were made from experience using a machine-smoothed-surface titanium implant. Publications by other investigators reported very high implant success rates in completely edentulous jaws, as well as predictable prosthetic reconstruction when the delayed loading protocol as advocated by Prof. Brånemark was followed. These articles were followed by publications indicating similar success rates with partially dentate cases.

The demands and expectations of patients to complete dental implant treatment sooner and faster have forced clinicians to find new clinical solutions. Fortunately, improvements in technology and understanding have provided the means for clinicians to meet these demands. Thus, with improvements in implant surfaces, thread patterns and implant body designs, loading concepts have evolved into the early loading of implants. Early loading is the application of load on implants sooner than the 3- to 6-month healing period, and immediate loading is the application of load within 48 hours. Early and immediate loading of dental implants requires clinicians to change their procedural protocols and patient management. To optimize treatment for their patients, clinicians must take advantage of all available improved technologies and clinical techniques, including CAD/CAM-generated surgical templates and prosthetic restorations, computer software programs that permit accurate diagnosis and treatment planning, and the use of minimally invasive surgical and prosthodontic techniques.

This textbook introduces the concept of NobelGuide, a complete and practical approach to managing the implant patient who expects immediate loading and function. The authors take the reader through the diagnostic process, with a detailed description of the necessary workup and generation of the radiographic guide for a CAT scan. This allows the clinician to complete the workup using a specialized computer software program that shows the available hard and soft tissues, vital anatomic structures and ideal locations for tooth/implant positions based on the prosthetic design. From this planning stage, a surgical template is generated for implant placement, allowing minimally invasive surgical techniques while assuring accuracy of implant placement without the reflection of a soft tissue flap. With knowledge of implant positions prior to the surgical placement, the prosthodontic specialist can fabricate the desired prosthesis before the actual surgery, thus providing the patient with a functioning prosthesis immediately after the implants are placed.

These new concepts and protocols are presented in a manner that allows clinicians to provide their patients with practical and predictable immediate function.

Editors

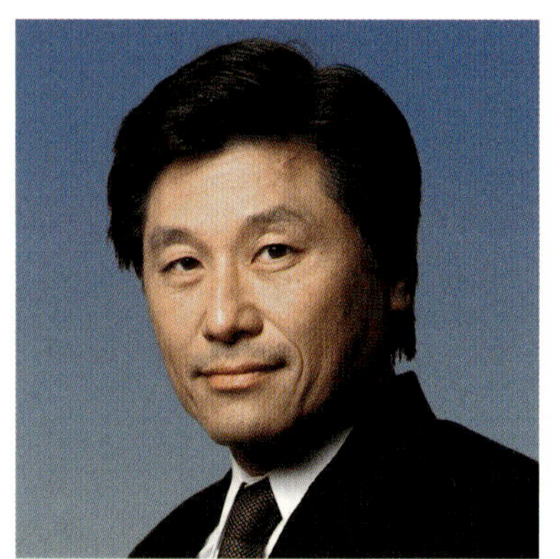
Peter K Moy

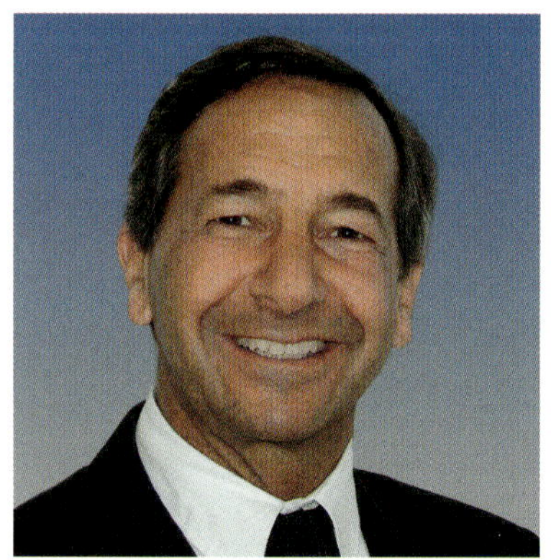
Patrick Palacci

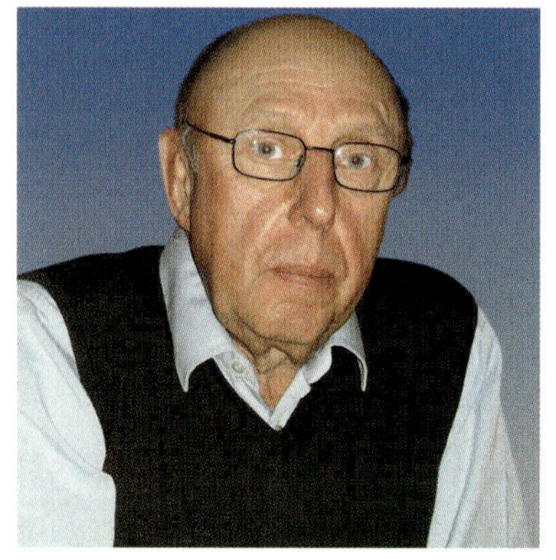
Ingvar Ericsson

Peter K Moy, DMD

Dr Moy received his dental degree from the University of Pittsburgh, a certificate in General Practice Residency from Queen's Medical Center in Honolulu, Hawaii, and completed his surgical training in oral and maxillofacial surgery at UCLA Hospital in 1982. A Professor in the Department of Oral and Maxillofacial Surgery at UCLA, he is also Director of Implant Dentistry at the Straumann Surgical Dental Center and Nobel Biocare Surgical Fellow Program. He is a Fellow of Pierre Fauchard Academy and the Academy of Osseointegration, where he currently serves as Vice President. He is an associate editor for the *International Journal of Oral and Maxillofacial Implants* and a member of the editorial board for the *International Journal of Oral and Maxillofacial Surgery*, *Clinical Implant Dentistry & Related Research* and *Oral Surgery, Oral Medicine, Oral Pathology, Oral Radiology and Endodontology*. Dr Moy maintains his private practice, the West Coast Oral & Maxillofacial Surgery Center, in Brentwood, California.

11980 San Vincente Blvd #503
Los Angeles CA 90049
USA
Tel: 001 310 820 6691
e-mail: drmoy@titaniumimplant.com

Patrick Palacci, DDS

Dr Palacci received his dental degree from the University of Marseilles, France; he completed his periodontal training at Boston University, MA, USA, where he was appointed as a Visiting Professor. He is currently in private practice at the Brånemark Osseointegration Center, Marseilles, which has mainly been involved in esthetic implant treatment, developing several techniques related to precision in osseointegration treatment as well as soft tissue management, including the papilla regeneration technique. He has written a number of scientific articles as well as two textbooks, published by Quintessence, and a chapter related to esthetics and soft tissue management in Professor Per-Ingvar Brånemark's textbook 'From Calvarium to Calcaneus', also published by Quintessence.

Brånemark Osseointegration Center
8-10 rue Fargès
13008 Marseilles
France
Tel: 00 33 (4) 91 57 03 03
e-mail: patrick@palacci.com

Ingvar Ericsson, DDS, Odont PhD

Prof Ericsson obtained his DDS degree in 1966; Specialist License in Periodontology in 1977, in Prosthetic Dentistry in 1990; and Odont doctorate degree (PhD) in 1978 at the Faculty of Odontology, Göteborg University, Sweden. He worked at the Department of Periodontology in Göteborg from 1973 to 1994, and as Professor at the Prosthodontic Department, Malmö University, from 1994 to 2003. In addition, he has been working as a private practitioner in Göteborg since 1967 and as a consultant at Nobel Biocare since 1993. Prof. Ericsson has published around 100 original articles, 25 review articles and several chapters in textbooks. He has been an invited speaker at approximately 200 scientific meetings and presented courses internationally. Prof. Ericsson has vast experience of the Brånemark System both from a surgical and a prosthetic point of view. He has been one of the clinical developers of the 'Teeth-in-an-Hour' concept, together with the group under Dr Matts Andersson at Nobel Biocare.

Djupedalsgatan 2
S-413 07 Gothenburg
Sweden
Tel: 00 46 707 615044
e-mail: the_iericsson@hotmail.com

Contents

Chapter 1

Loading principles

Ingvar Ericsson

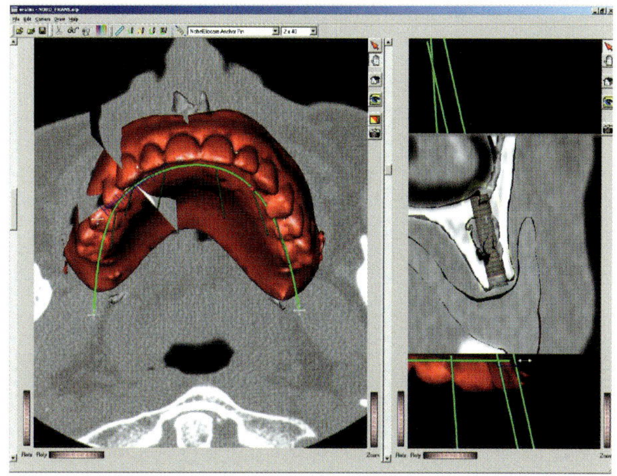

Delayed, early and immediate loading protocol

Two-stage surgery – delayed loading

In 1969, the original protocol for implant installation was described by Brånemark and co-workers (Brånemark et al 1969). The protocol specifies a two-stage surgical procedure, i.e. a two-piece implant is used and the implant is submerged during a 3- to 6-month healing period (Fig 1-1). Thereafter, abutment connection is performed, the supra-construction fabricated and screw-retained to the implant pillars. The principle of osseointegration was emphasized: '...direct anchorage of an implant by the formation of bony tissue at the bone implant interface as observed at the light microscopic level'.

In 1977, follow-up results of the treatment outcome of 235 edentulous jaws (128 maxillas and 107 mandibles) were presented (Brånemark et al 1977). The observation period varied from 9 months to 8 years. Data revealed that 85% of all the supra-constructions installed were stable. Since then, a high predictability of implant treatment has been demonstrated in long-term follow-up studies (5–15 years) for edentulous patients (e.g. Adell et al 1990, Arvidsson et al 1996, 1998) and for partially dentate patients (e.g. Lekholm et al 1999). Therefore, the implant methodology has a scientific foundation for implant stability and predictable long-term clinical success.

One-stage surgery – delayed loading

The Brånemark System for implants was originally designed to be a two-stage system: during the initial healing phase the implants were submerged. This approach was taken to minimize risk of infection, prevent apical migration of mucosal epithelium along the titanium surface and to minimize the risk for undue early loading of the implant (Brånemark et al 1969, 1977).

However, since its development, there has been a re-evaluation of the traditional two-stage protocol. Schroeder et al (1976, 1978, 1983) showed that it is possible to achieve predictable osseointegration even when using a one-stage technique, i.e. immediately following installation, the implant pillar is exposed in the oral cavity. In experimental studies, the application of a one-stage surgical procedure of one-piece implants (Gotfredsen et al 1991, Abrahamsson et al 1996) or two-piece implants (Abrahamsson et al 1996, Ericsson et al 1996) has shown good results. These observations are further confirmed in a number of well-controlled clinical studies using the Brånemark System (e.g. Henry and Rosenberg 1994, Bernard et al 1995, Becker et al 1997, Ericsson et al 1997, Collært and De Bruyn 1998, Friberg et al 1999, Bogærde et al 2003, Rocci et al 2003a, Engquist et al 2005). Furthermore, Ericsson et al (1997) reported that the marginal bone level at turned implants placed anteriorly in the edentulous mandible, and supporting fixed supra-constructions, is stable between 12 and 60 months, irrespective of whether placed according to a one- or two-stage surgical protocol.

Becker et al (1997) reported on 135 Brånemark turned implants placed according to the one-stage surgical protocol in combination with delayed loading (i.e. 3–6 months of healing before loading; Fig 1-1). Implants were placed in the maxilla as well as in the mandible, demonstrating partially dentate conditions. The implant survival rate during the first year of observation following loading was 95–96%. A noteworthy finding was that in this particular group of patients, 32 single tooth replacements were included (Becker et al 1997).

Collært and De Bruyn (1998) treated 85 patients for partial (n = 35) or complete (n = 50) mandibular edentulousness by means of fixed supra-constructions retained by Brånemark turned implants. A total of 330 implant pillars were placed. Of these 330 implants, 211 were installed according to the one-stage protocol (i.e. 3–4 months of healing before loading) and 119 according to the traditional two-stage protocol. A somewhat higher percentage of failures was reported for the partially situation than for the completely edentulous situation, irrespective of whether the implants were placed using a one- or two-stage surgical approach. The overall implant survival rate, during the up to 2-year observation period, was reported to be about 95%. The authors concluded that '... a one-

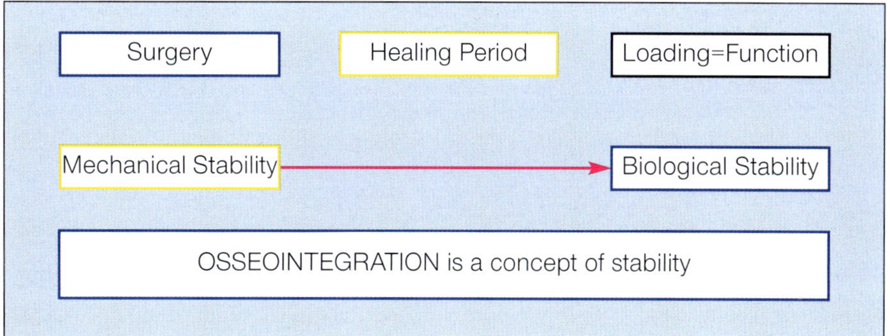

Fig 1-1 Schematic illustration of the two-stage and one-stage surgical protocol with delayed loading.

stage surgical approach with normally submerged-type Brånemark implants can be as predictable as the common two-stage procedure in the completely and partially edentulous mandible'.

Hermans and co-workers (1977) treated 13 patients for edentulism in the mandible using implants placed in a one-stage surgical procedure. The follow-up period was 3 years and '... the cumulative failure rate reached for the single step operative technique was 1.9%'. In other words, a similar treatment outcome was obtained for the one-stage technique as for the traditional submerged one. Bernard et al (1995) placed 10 implants according to a one-stage surgical technique in five edentulous mandibles. Following the initial 3-month healing period, the implants served as retainers for overdentures. No implant failure, either peri-implant soft or hard tissue complication, was reported.

Similar clinical data have been reported with use of ITI implants (one-piece) in different situations (Buser et al 1997): in edentulous mandibles (Hellem et al 2001), and in edentulous maxillas (Bergkvist et al 2004). In these clinical studies, the implant pillars were not loaded via a fixed supraconstruction until 3 to 6 months of healing had passed. In other words, the treatment concept of one-stage implant installation in combination with delayed loading was applied (Fig 1-1). Furthermore, data from clinical studies using Astra Tech implants (two-piece) support the above-mentioned observations (e.g. Cooper et al 1999).

In all the clinical studies cited above, the original dentures most often were adjusted and relined by a soft tissue conditioner 1–2 weeks following implant installation to minimize unfavorable functional loading of the implants. However, it should be anticipated that implants installed according to a one-stage surgical procedure during the initial healing period, to some extent, will be directly and unpredictably loaded during function via the adjusted and relined denture. Furthermore, such loading might be unfavorable for the implants, as the deformation pattern of complete denture base material during functional conditions can be complex and unpredictable (Glantz and Stafford 1983). Despite this, Brånemark turned implants installed according to a one-stage surgical procedure demonstrated the same successful rate as identical implants installed according to the original two-stage procedure (e.g. Ericsson et al 1994, 1997, Bernard et al 1995, Becker et al 1997a, Hermans et al 1997, Collært and De Bruyn 1998). In other words, '... an initial and direct loading of implants piercing the mucosa via the adjusted and relined denture obviously does not jeopardize a proper osseointegration of the fixtures' (Ericsson et al 1997). Such a statement is in agreement with clinical data reported by Henry and Rosenberg (1994), who concluded that: '... controlled immediate loading of adequately installed, non-submerged implants, by reinsertion of a modified denture, does not appear to jeopardize the process of osseointegration in the anterior mandible'. Furthermore, Becker et al (1997) claimed that '... one-step Brånemark implants may be considered a viable alternative to two-step implants'. According to Glantz et al (1984a, 1984b), favorable loading

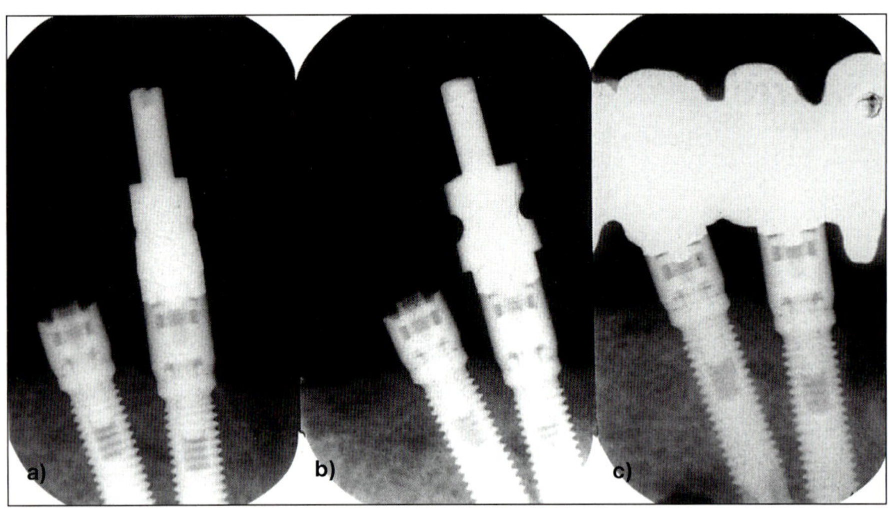

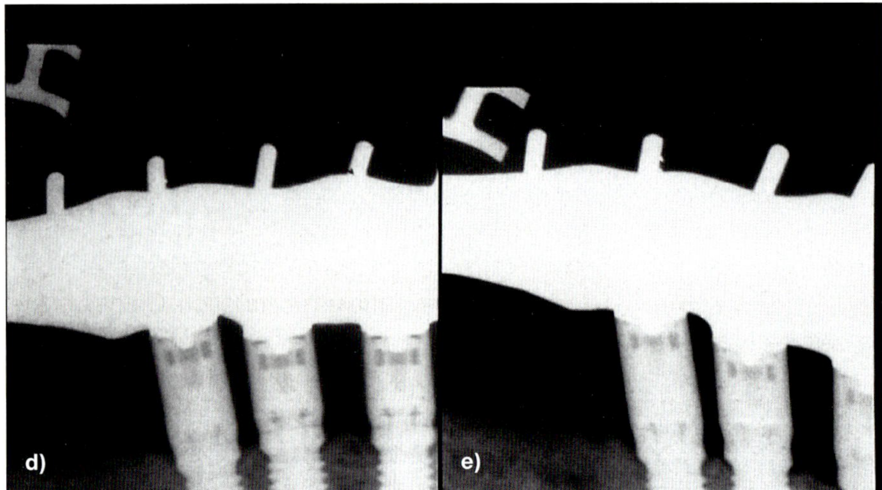

Fig 1-2 **(a–c)** Marginal bone level around implants placed according to the one-stage surgical protocol with early loading. **(a)** Condition at time of placement. **(b)** At 18-months' follow-up. **(c)** At 60-month follow-up examination. **(d and e)** Marginal bone level around implants placed and loaded according to the original protocol: **(d)** condition at 18-months' follow-up examination, and **(e)** at 5-year follow-up examinaton.

conditions are achieved through a rigid fixed supraconstruction and, therefore, it is reasonable to believe that a successful treatment outcome could be reached also when rigid appliances are connected to the turned implants early following installation of the implants (i.e. early functional loading).

The importance of oral hygiene has been highlighted, especially when applying the one-stage surgical protocol (Gotfredsen et al 1991). Good oral hygiene conditions will facilitate the formation of a proper soft tissue sealant, i.e. the tissue portion separating the oral cavity and the anchoring bone. The authors concluded that plaque accumulation on the implant pillars resulted in: (1) extended infiltrated connective tissue, not only in a vertical but also in a horizontal direction; (2) long pocket epithelium; and (3) active bone resorption (i.e. presence of osteoclasts) of the marginal bone crest compared with the conditions at implants without presence of plaque accumulations.

One-stage surgery – early loading

About 20 years ago, it was stated that '... premature load on implants leads to the formation of fibrous tissue instead of the formation of bone tissue' (i.e. ontogenesis; Albrektsson et al 1986). When implants are placed according to the one-stage protocol, the implants most likely will be exposed to a certain load immediately following placement.

An important prerequisite for obtaining a predictable healing process of implants (osseointegration) is that 'micromotion' (i.e. the movement at the interface between the bone and the implant

Fig 1-3 Treatment approach by Schnitman and co-workers (1997). Five to six implants were placed in the anterior mandible between the foramina, and one of these implants close to the midline was exposed to abutment connection immediately following installation. Remaining implants were submerged and abutments were connected 3 to 4 months later. In addition, distal to the exit of and above the nerve-vessel bundle, one short implant was placed bilaterally using a one-stage surgical technique. Thus three implants were exposed in the oral cavity, which were immediately connected to an interim fixed partial denture. Three to four months later, the permanent fixed partial denture was fabricated and attached to all available implants.

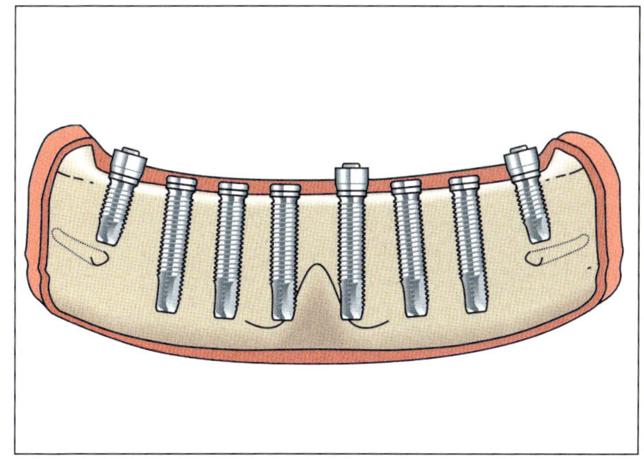

surface) is limited (Cameron et al 1973, Brunski 1992, 1999, Pilliar 1995). Søballe et al (1993) reported that the tissues involved probably will accept micromotion amounting to 50–150 µm. Furthermore, Brunski (1999) reported that micromotion of approximately 100 µm may constitute a threshold value for turned implant surfaces to osseointegrate properly.

Favorable loading conditions can be achieved for teeth connected to each other via a rigid fixed partial denture (Glantz et al 1984a, 1984b). However, individual implant pillars installed according to the one-stage surgical procedure are most likely exposed to unpredictable load immediately after installation. Therefore, it is reasonable to assume that implants have to be joined together via a rigid construction as soon as possible following placement. Micromotion at the interface between bone and implant surfaces will be limited and, hopefully, within an acceptable level, thus facilitating the healing process (osseointegration).

Recently, good and predictable results of implant treatment have been reported in the literature when implants are exposed to early functional load in the anterior mandible (e.g. Ericsson et al 2000, Chow et al 2001, Friberg et al 2005). Thus, Ericsson et al (2000) evaluated the outcome of oral rehabilitations of edentulous mandibles by fixed supra-constructions connected to turned Brånemark implants installed according to either (1) a one-stage surgical procedure and immediate loading, or (2) the original two-stage delayed loading protocol – with the working hypothesis that there is no difference between the two methods concerning the treatment outcome. A total of 88 turned implants (16 patients) were placed according to the one-stage protocol and loaded via a fixed appliance within 20 days. Implants placed according to the original protocol were loaded about 4 months following implant installation. On delivery of the fixed appliances, all patients were radiographically examined; this examination was repeated at 18- and 60-months' follow ups. Analysis of the radiographs revealed that, during the entire observation period, the mean loss of bone support amounted to less than 1.0 mm around the implants irrespective of whether early loaded or not (Fig 1-2). All implants at all observation intervals were found to be clinically stable. The authors concluded that it is '... possible to successfully load titanium dental implants early following installation via a permanent fixed rigid cross-arch supra-construction'.

Recently, Friberg et al (2005) reported a retrospective study. The purpose was to evaluate the 1-year results of one-stage surgery and early loading in a large group of patients. Data obtained were compared with those of a study from the same clinic, applying the original protocol (i.e. two-stage and delayed loading). The authors concluded as follows: '... the present investigation showed a high but (compared with the classic two-stage technique) somewhat lower cumulative survival rate (CSR) after 1 year for the one-stage technique' (CSR: 97.5% vs 99.7%, respectively).

One-stage surgery – immediate loading

Schnitman and co-workers (1997) reported on 63 Brånemark turned implants placed in 10 patients (Fig 1-3). Of these 63 implants, 28 were placed and ' ... immediately loaded to support an interim fixed bridge'. Of these 28 implants, four failed. The remaining 35 implants installed according to the original two-stage protocol all osseointegrated properly. In other words, the survival rate for the immediately loaded implants was about 85%. However, it should be noted that Schnitman et al (1997) reported on a 10-year outcome. The survival rate for the submerged implants was 100%. Furthermore, Balshi and Wolfinger (1997) applied a treatment approach for the edentulous mandible similar to that of Schnitman and co-workers. They reported that 80% (32 of 40) of the immediately loaded Brånemark implants survived over the observation period. They concluded that '... preliminary results have been favorable, with all patients functioning with a fixed implant prosthesis from the day of first-stage surgery'.

Another treatment modality has recently been presented, namely the 'Brånemark Novum' concept (Brånemark et al 1999). 'The new protocol involves prefabricated components and surgical guides, elimination of the prosthetic impression procedure, and attachment of the permanent bridge on the day of implant placement.' Fifty patients were followed 6 months to 3 years after completion of the rehabilitation. Three implants failed to integrate and three implants were lost during the observation period, resulting in an overall survival rate of 98% and a prosthetic survival rate also of 98%. The average bone loss is in agreement with figures reported for the original protocol and '... did not exceed 0.2 mm per year when calculated from the 3-month examination'. Furthermore, van Steenberghe et al (2004) reported on 50 patients treated according to the Brånemark Novum concept with follow-up over a 12-month period. The cumulative success rate for implants and prostheses was found to be 93% and 95% respectively, thus supporting the data presented by Brånemark et al (1999).

In 2001, Hatano presented the 'Maxis New' technique, another one-day treatment of the edentulous mandible using standard Brånemark System components and an individualized fixed partial denture (Hatano 2001). The author concluded: '... the treatment was successful in 35 patients followed for 2 to 36 months of loading'.

Soon after, a report was published on an 18-month clinical follow-up study to compare the treatment outcome of TiUnite and turned-surfaced Brånemark System implants when applying immediate loading via cross-arch-designed fixed partial dentures in the anterior mandible (Fröberg et al 2006). Fifteen patients with edentulous mandibles participated. In one half of the jaw, between the exit of the nerve–vessel bundle and the midline, one type of implant was placed, and in the remaining half the other type. The 89 implants (44 TiUnite™ and 45 turned, respectively) were loaded the day of surgery via a fixed, temporary supra-construction. Ten days later, the permanent one was screw-retained to the implant pillars. The authors concluded that: '... a high predictability regarding the treatment outcome for immediately loaded Brånemark implants in the anterior mandible was observed. Furthermore, no difference between the traditional turned and the an-oxidized implant surface (TiUnite™) could be observed. However, it has to be stressed that all implants (irrespective of surface) were placed in the anterior mandible and also that all patients demonstrated a high level of oral hygiene.' In general, it should be emphasized that the immediate splinting of the implants most likely is of utmost importance for the high cumulative survival rate reported (Fig 1-4).

To challenge the original protocol for Brånemark System implant installation further, a study was designed to evaluate the treatment outcome using the one-stage protocol and immediate loading for single crown restorations (Ericsson et al 2001). Fourteen patients were treated according to the following protocol: after placement of the turned implant, an impression was immediately taken and a temporary crown in light central occlusion and with no lateral load contacts was fabricated and connected within 24 hours. Three to six months later, the temporary crown was replaced by a permanent one. During the same period, eight patients with single tooth loss were treated accord-

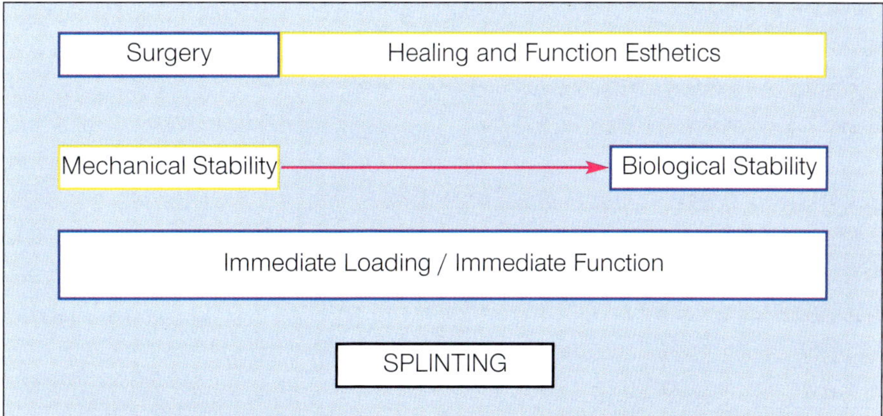

Fig 1-4 One-stage early and immediate loading protocol emphasizing the importance of splinting.

ing to the standard protocol. These patients served as controls. Radiographs were taken at the 6-, 18- and 60-month follow-up examination. Two implants that were immediately loaded were lost during the observation period (3 and 5 months following placement, respectively; cumulative survival rate 85%), and a similar mean loss of supporting bone (about 0.1 mm) was observed in this group of patients compared with a control group treated according to the traditional protocol. Therefore, the marginal bone level changes observed are in agreement with figures reported earlier (e.g. Brånemark et al 1999, Ericsson et al 2001, van Steenberghe et al 2004), which lends further support to the feasibility to apply such a treatment approach for single tooth restorations. However, it should be noted that in the studies citied traditional turned implants were used. Clinical trials using implants with a rougher surface have shown a better treatment outcome. Thus, Maló et al (2003) and Calendriello and Tomatis (2004) used TiUnite implants for single tooth restorations (immediately loaded) and showed a cumulative survival rate amounting to around 98%. Similar data have been reported by Kirketerp et al (2002) using Replace Select HA-coated implants installed and loaded immediately following extraction (see Fig 1-5).

During the introduction of the osseointegration concept (Brånemark et al 1969), there was increased interest in the texture and condition of the implant surfaces. Implant surface can vary significantly depending on its preparation and handling (Kasemo and Lausmaa 1988). It is generally accepted that the outermost atomic layer of the implant surfaces is a key factor for the osseointegration process. The cell–oxide interaction takes place over a few atomic distances; compositional changes occurring at that level could influence biocompatibility and healing (Kasemo and Lausmaa 1985). Currently, it is generally accepted that implants with a somewhat rough surface will (1) facilitate initial stability, (2) enlarge the surface area (Wennerberg 1996) and (3) speed up osseointegration (Larsson 2000, Schüpbach et al 2005). Thus the issue of surface characteristics has

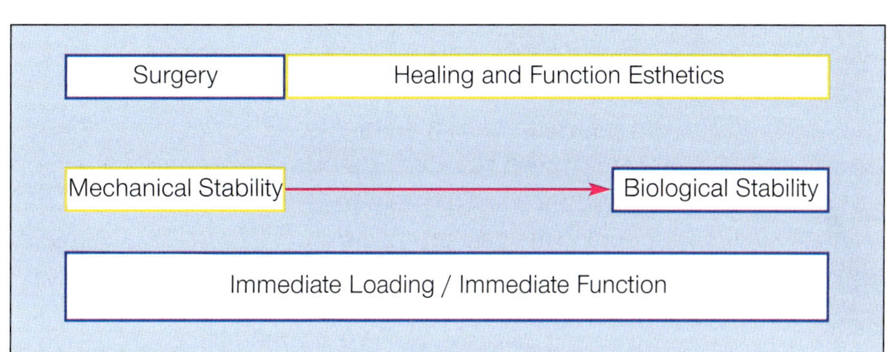

Fig 1-5 Schematic illustration of the one-stage early and immediate loading protocol.

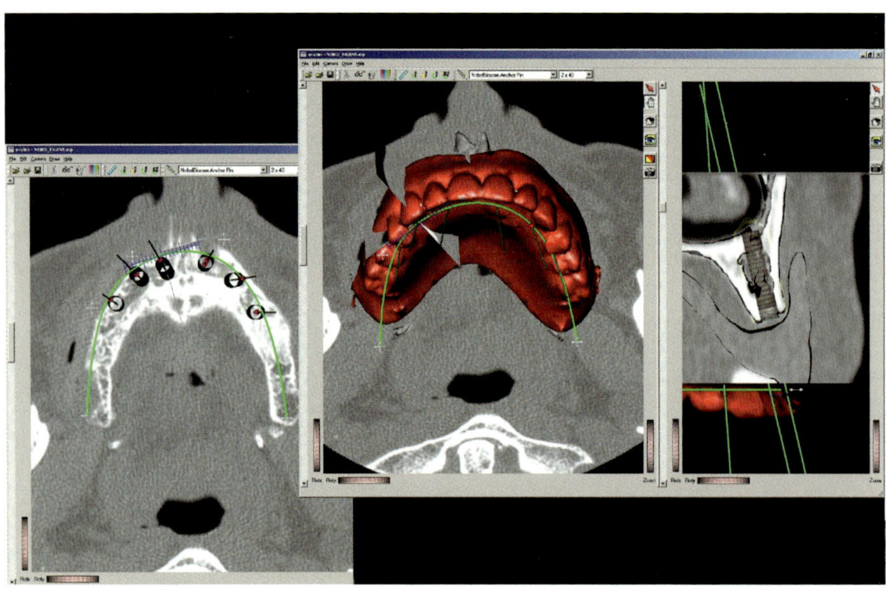

Fig 1-6 Virtual planning procedure: three-dimensional (left and middle) and two-dimensional (right).

gained prominence (Karlsson et al 1998, Cordioli et al 2000, Gotfredsen et al 2000, Gotfredsen and Karlsson 2001). To create such a surface, the clinician can, for example, blast it, apply titanium plasma spray, or perform an anodic oxidation of the surface (Hall and Lausmaa 2000). Experimental studies have shown that the bone-to-implant contact is higher for a TiUnite™ (anoxidized [anodically oxidized]) surface compared with a machined one (Albrektsson et al 2000, Henry et al 2000, Rocci et al 2003b, Zechner et al 2003); an observation which is in agreement with human histological findings recently reported (Rocci et al 2002, Ivanoff et al 2003, Schüpbach et al 2005). This is possibly due to osteoconductive properties of the TiUnite™ surface. In addition, Rompen et al (2000) demonstrated, using a dog model, that an-oxidized (TiUnite™) implants will maintain their primary stability better than machined ones. This observation is supported by clinical data reported by Glauser et al. (2001). Therefore, it seems reasonable to state that TiUnite implants are well suited to exposure to immediate functional load. In other words, a paradigm shift has occurred regarding the loading concept of dental implants. Today, it is not only possible to load the implants the day of installation via a rigid, provisional supra-construction, but also to fabricate the final one before placing the implants (NobelGuide concept). By using spiral computerized tomography, converted scanning data and an advanced virtual planning program, it is possible to '... place the implants in their best position in the jawbone' before the real surgery is performed (Fig 1-6). This book will deal with this topic of virtual planning for implant surgery.

References

Abrahamsson I, Berglundh T, Wennström J, Lindhe J. The peri-implant hard and soft tissues at different implant systems. A comparative study in the dog. Clin Oral Implants Res 1996;7:212-219.

Adell R, Eriksson B, Lekholm U, Brånemark P-I, Jemt T. A long-term follow-up study of osseointegrated implants in the treatment of totally edetulous jaws. Int J Oral Maxillofac Implants 1990;5:347-359.

Albrektsson T, Zarb G, Worthington P, Eriksson RA. The long-term efficacy of currently used dental implants: a review and proposed criteria of success. Int J Oral Maxillofac Implants 1986;1:11–25.

Albrektsson T, Johansson C, Lundgren AK, Sul Y, Gottlow J, Experimental studies on oxidized implant. A histomorphometrical and biomechanical analysis. Appl Osseointegration Res 2000;1:21-24.

Arvidson K, Bystedt H, Frykholm A et al. Five-year follow-up report of the Astra Dental Implant system for restoration of edentulous upper jaws. J Dent Res 1996;75:349(Abstract).

Arvidson K, Bystedt H, Frykholm A, Konow L, Lothigus E. Five-year prospective follow-up report of the Astra Tech Dental Implant System in the treatment of edentulous mandibles. Clin Oral Implants Res 1998;9:225–234.

Balshi TJ, Wolfinger GJ. Immediate loading of Brånemark implants in edentulous mandibles: a preliminary report. Implant Dent 1997;6:83-88.

Becker W, Becker BE, Isrælson H, Lucchini JP, Handelsman M, Ammons W. One-step surgical placement of Brånemark implants: a prospective clinical multicenter study. Int J Oral Maxillofac Implants 1997;12:454-462.

Bergkvist G, Sahlholm S, Nilner K, Lindh C. Implant-supported fix prostheses in the edentulous maxilla. A 2-year clinical and radiological follow-up of treatment with non-submerged ITI implants. Clin Oral Implants Res 2004;15:351-359.

Bernard J-P, Belser UC, Martinet J-P, Borgis SA. Osseointegration of Brånemark fixtures using a single-step operating technique. A preliminary prospective one-year study in the edentulous mandible. Clin Oral Implants Res 1995;6:122-129.

Bogærde L, Padretti G, Dellacasa P, Mozzati M, Rangert B, Eng M. Early function of splinted implants in maxillas and posterior mandibles using Brånemark System, machined-surface implant: an 18 month prospective multicenter study. Clin Implant Dent Relat Res 2003;5(Suppl 1):21-28.

Brunski JE. Biomechanical factors affecting the bone–dental implant interface. Clin Mater 1992;3:153-201.

Brunski JE. *In vivo* bone response to biomechanical loading at the bone/dental implant interface. Adv Dent Res 1999;13:99-119.

Brånemark P-I, Breine U, Adel R, Hansson B-O, Ohlsson Å. Intra-osseous anchorage of dental procthoses. I. Experimental studies. Scand J Plast Reconstr Surg 1969;3:81-100.

Brånemark P-I, Hansson BO, Adell R et al. Osseointegrated implants in the treatment of the edentulous jaw. Experience from a 10-year period. Scand J Plast Reconstr Surg Suppl 1977;11:16:1-32.

Brånemark P-I, Engstrand P, Öhrnell L-O et al. Brånemark Novum: A new treatment concept for rehabilitation of the edentulous mandible. Preliminary results from a prospective clinical follow-up study. Clin Implant Dent Relat Res 1999;1:2-16.

Buser D, Mericske-Stern R, Bernard JP, Behneke N, Hirt HP, Belser UC et al. Long-term evaluation of non-submerged ITI implants. Part I: 8-year life table analysis of a prospective multicenter study with 2359 implants. Clin Oral Implants Res 1997;8:161-172.

Calandriello R, Tomatis M. Immediate function of single implants using Brånemark System: prospective one year report of final restorations. Appl Osseointegration Res 2004;4:32-40.

Cameron H, Pilliar RM, Macnab I. The effect of movement on the bonding of porous metal to bone. J Biomed Mater Res 1973;7:301-311.

Chow J, Hui E, Li D, Liu J. Immediate loading of Brånemark system fixtures in the mandible with a fixed provisional prothesis. Appl Osseointergration Res 2001;2:30-35.

Collært B, De Bruyn H. Comparison of Brånemark fixture integration and short-term survival using one-stage or two-stage surgery in completely and partially edentulous mandibles. Clin Oral Implants Res 1998;9:131-135.

Cooper LF, Scurria MS, Lang LA, Guckes AD, Moriarty JD, Felton DA. Treatment of edentulism using Astra Tech implants and ball abutments to retain mandibular overdentures. Int J Oral Maxillofac Implants 1999;14:646-653.

Cordioli G, Majzoub Z, Piattelli A, Scarano ATI. Removal torque and histomorphometric investigation of 4 different titanium surfaces: an experimental study in the rabbit tibia. Int J Oral Maxillofac Implants 2000;15:668-674.

Engquist B, Åstrand P, Anzén B, Dahlgren S, Enquist E, Feldman H. Simplified methods of implant treatment in the edentulous lower jaw: a 3-year follow-up report of a controlled prospective study of one-stage versus two-stage surgery and early loading. Clin Implant Dent Relat Res 2005;7:95-104

Ericsson I, Randow K, Glantz P-O, Lindhe J, Nilner K. Some clinical and radiographical features of submerged and non-submerged titanium implants. Clin Oral Implants Res 1994;5:185-189.

Ericsson I, Nilner K, Klinge B, Glantz P-O. Radiographical and histological characteristics of submerged and non-submerged titanium implants. An experimental study in the Labrador dog. Clin Oral Implants Res 1996;6:20-26.

Ericsson I, Randow K, Nilner K, Petersson A. Some clinical and radiographical features of submerged and non-submerged titanium implants. A 5-year follow-up study. Clin Oral Implants Res 1997;8:422-426.

Ericsson I, Randow K, Nilner K, Petersson A. Early functional loading of Brånemark dental implants. A 5-year follow-up study. Clin Implant Dent Relat Res 2000;2:70-77.

Ericsson I, Nilson H, Nilner K. Immediate functional loading of Brånemark single tooth implants. A 5-year clinical follow-up study. Appl Osseointegration Res 2001;2:12-16.

Friberg B, Sennerby L, Lindén B, Gröndahl K, Lekholm U. Stability measurements of one-stage Brånemark implants during healing in mandibles. A clinical resonance frequency analysis study. Int J Oral Maxillofac Surg 1999;28:266-272.

Friberg B, Henningsson C, Jemt T. Rehabilitation of edentulous mandibles by means of turned Brånemark System implants after one-stage surgery: a 1-year retrospective study of 152 patients. Clin Implant Dent Relat Res 2005;7:1-9.

Fröberg KK, Lindh C, Ericsson I. Immediate loading of Brånemark System implants: a comparison between TiUnite and turned implants placed in the anterior mandible. Clin Implant Dent Relat Res 2006;8:187-197.

Glantz P-O, Stafford GD. Clinical deformation of maxillary complete dentures. J Dent 1983;11:224-230.

Glantz P-O, Strandman E, Svensson SA, Randow K. On functional strain in fixed mandibular reconstructions. I. An *in vitro* study. Acta Odontol Scand 1984a; 42:241-249.

Glantz P-O, Strandman E, Randow K. On functional strain in fixed mandibular reconstructions. II. An *in vivo* study. Acta Odontol Scand 1984b;42:269-276.

Glauser R, Portmann M, Ruhstaller P, Lundgren A-K, Hämmerle CHF, Gottlow J. Stability measurements of immediately loaded machined and oxidized implants in the posterior maxilla. A comparative clinical study using resonance frequency analysis. Appl Osseointegration Res 2001;2:27-29.

Gotfredsen K, Rostrup E, Hjorting-Hansen E, Stoltz K, Budtz-Jörgensen E. Histological and histomorphometric evaluation of tissue reactions adjacent to endosteal implants in monkeys. Clin Oral Implants Res 1991;2:30-37.

Gotfredsen K, Berglundh T, Lindhe J. Anchorage of titanium

implants with different surface characteristics: an experimental study in rabbits. Clin Implant Dent Relat Res 2000;2:70-77.
Gotfredsen K, Karlsson U. A prospective 5-year study of fixed partial prosthesis supported by implants with machined and TiO_2- blasted surface. J Prosthodontics 2001;10:2-7.
Hall J, Lausmaa J. Properties of a new porous oxide surface on titanium implants. Appl Osseointegration Res 2000;1:5-8.
Hatano N. The Maxis New. A novel one-day technique for fixed individualized implant-supported prosthesis in the edentulous mandible using Brånemark System implants. Appl Osseointegration Res 2001;2:40-43.
Hellem S, Karlsson U, Almfelt I, Brunell SE, Åstrand P. Non-submerged implant in the treatment of the edentulous lower jaw: a 5-year prospective longitudinal study of ITI hollow screws. Clin Implant Dent Relat Res 2001;3:20-29.
Henry P, Rosenberg J. Single-stage surgery for rehabilitation of the edentulous mandible. Preliminary results. Pract Periodont Aesthet Dent 1994;6:1-8.
Henry P, Tan A, Allen B, Hall J, Johansson C. Removal torque comparison of TiUnite and turned implants in the greyhound dog mandible. Appl Osseointegration Res 2000;1:15-17.
Hermans M, Durdu F, Herrman I, Malevez C. A single-step operative technique using the Brånemark system. A prospective study in the edentulous mandible. Clin Oral Implants Res 1997;8:437(Abstract).
Ivanoff CJ, Widmark G, Johansson C, Wennerberg A. Histologic evaluation of bone response to oxidized and turned titanium micro-implants in human jawbone. Int J Oral Maxillofac Implants 2003;18:341-348.
Karlsson U, Gotfredsen K, Olsson C. A 2-year report on maxillary and mandibular fixed partial dentures supported by Astra Tech dental implants. A comparison of 2 implants. Clin Oral Implants Res 1998;9:235-242.
Kasemo B, Lausmaa J. Aspects of surface physics on titanium implants. Swed Dent J 1985;28(Suppl):19-36.
Kasemo B, Lausmaa J. Biomaterial and implant surface science: a surface science approach. Int J Oral Maxillofac Implants 1988;4:247-259.
Kirketerp P, Andersen J, Urde G. Replacement of extracted anterior teeth by immediately loaded Replace Select HA-coated implants. An one-year follow-up of 35 patients. Appl Osseointegration Res 2002;3:40-43.
Larsson C. The interface between bone and implants with different surface oxide properties. Appl Osseointegration Res 2000;1:9-14.
Lekholm U, Gunne J, Henry P, Higuchi K, Lindén U, Bergström C. Survival of the Brånemark implant in partially edentulous jaws: a 10-year prospective multicenter study. Int J Oral Maxillofac Implants 1999;14:639-645.
Maló P, Friberg B, Polozzi G, Gualini F, Vighagen T, Rangert B. Immediate and early function of Brånemark implants placed in the esthetic zone: a 1-year prospective clinical multicenter study. Clin Implant Dent Relat Res 2003;5(Suppl 1):37-46.
Pilliar RM. Quantitative evaluation of the effect of movement at a porous coated implant-bone interface. In: Davies EJ (ed). The bone–biomaterial interface. Toronto: University of Toronto Press, 1995;380-387.
Rocci A, Martignoni M, Sennerby L, Gottlow J. Immediate loading of a Brånemark System implant with the TiUnite surface. Histological evaluation after 9 months. Appl Osseointegration Res 2002;3:25-28.
Rocci A, Martignoni M, Burgos PM, Gottlow J, Sennerby L. Histology of retrieved immediately and early loaded oxidized implants: light microscopic observations after 5 to 9 months of loading in the posterior mandible. Clin Implant Dent Relat Res 2003a;5(Suppl 1):88-98.
Rocci A, Martignoni M, Gottlow J. Immediate loading of Brånemark system with TiUnite and machined surfaces in the posterior mandible: a randomized, open-ended trial. Clin Implant Dent Relat Res 2003b;5(Suppl 1):57-63
Rompen E, DaSilva D, Lundgren AK, Gottlow J, Sennerby L. Stability measurements of a double-threaded titanium implant design with turned or oxidized surface. An experimental resonance frequency analysis study in the dog mandible. Appl Osseointegration Res 2000;1:18-20.
Schnitman PA, Wöhrle PS, Rubenstein JE, Da Silva JD, Wang N-H. Ten year results for Brånemark implants immediately loaded with fixed prostheses at implant placement. Int J Oral Maxillofac Implants 1997; 12:495-503.
Schroeder A, Pohler O, Sutter F. Gewebsreaktion auf ein Titan-Hohlzylinder-Implantat mit Titan-Spritz-schichtoberfäche. Schweiz Monatschr Zahnheilkd 1976;86:713-727.
Schroder A, Stich H, Straumann F, Sutter F. Über die Anlagerung Osteocement an einem belasteten Implantatkörper. Schweiz Monatschr Zahnheilk 1978;88:1051-1058.
Schroder A, Mæglin B, Sutter F. Das ITI-Hohlzylinderimplantat Typ F zur Prothesenretention beim zahnlosen Kiefer. Schweiz Monatschr Zahnheilk 1983;93:720-733.
Schüpbach P, Glauser R, Rocci A, Martignani M, Sennerby L, Lundgren AK. The human bone-oxidized titanium implant interface: a light microscopic, scanning electron microscopic, black-scatter scanning electron microscopic, and energy-dispersive X-ray study of clinically retrieved dental implants. Clin Implant Dent Relat Res 2005;7(Suppl 1):36-43.
Søballe K, Hansen ES, Brockstedt-Rasmussen H, Bünger C. The effects of osteoporosis, bone deficiency, bone grafting and micromotion on fixation of porous-coated hydroxyapatite-coated implants. In: Gesink, RGT, Manley MT (eds). Hydroxypatite coatings in orthopædic surgery. New York: Raven Press, 1993;107-136.
van Steenberghe D, Molly L, Jacobs R, Vandekerckhove B, Quirynen M, Nært I. The immediate rehabilitation by means of a ready-made final fixed prosthesis in the edentulous mandible: a 1-year follow-up study of 50 consecutive patients. Clin Oral Implants Res 2004;15:360-365.
Wennerberg A. On surface roughness and implant incorporation [PhD thesis]. Department of Biomaterials/ Handicap Research, Göteborg University, Sweden, 1996.
Zechner W, Tangl S, Fürst G, Tepper G, Thams U, Mailath G. Osseous healing characteristics of three different implant types. A histological and histomorphometric study in mini-pigs. Clin Oral Implants Res 2003;14:150-157.

Chapter 2

NobelGuide concept

Peter K Moy

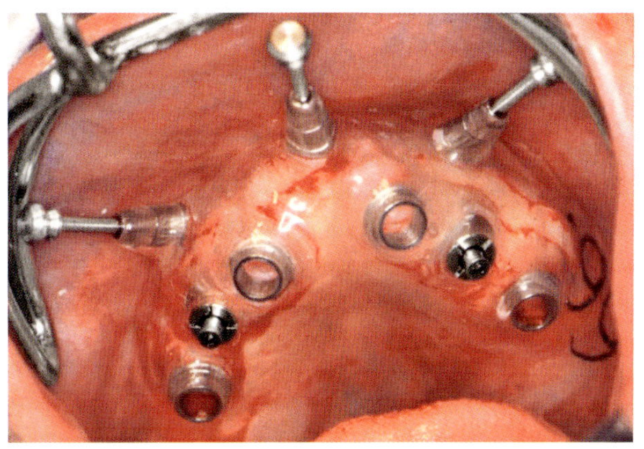

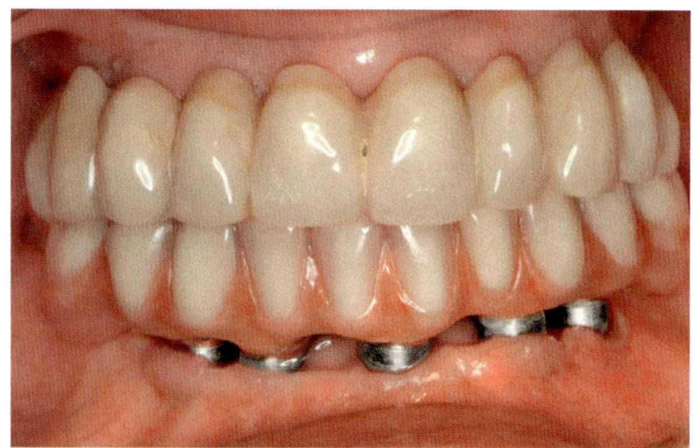

Fig 2-1 Fuctionally stable mandibular implant-supported prosthesis at 15-years.

Background

A conventional approach to osseointegration has proven to be highly successful (Brånemark et al 1977). Long-term stability with implants supporting a functioning prosthesis has been a clinical reality for well over 20 years (Fig 2-1). Many patients have benefited from the reliability of titanium dental implants and improved function, as well as improved esthetics of implant-supported restorations compared with conventional dental restorations. Clinicians have benefited also. With dental implants, they can restore any edentulous situation: from the completely edentulous patient, to the partially dentate, to the single-missing tooth (Fig 2-2). New surgical techniques have been developed to manage the more demanding, partially dentate situation with adverse alveolar contours in the esthetic zone (Glauser et al 2003).

As the clinician's ability to manage any clinical situation with dental implants has improved, the demand from patients for dental implants has increased. Completely edentulous and partially dentate patients wearing a removable prosthesis are requesting more stable, fixed restorations within a quicker time period than the typical 4 to 6 months of healing that was necessary with the

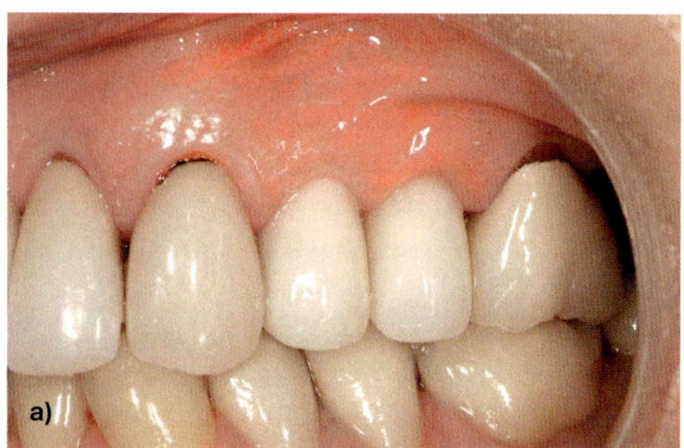

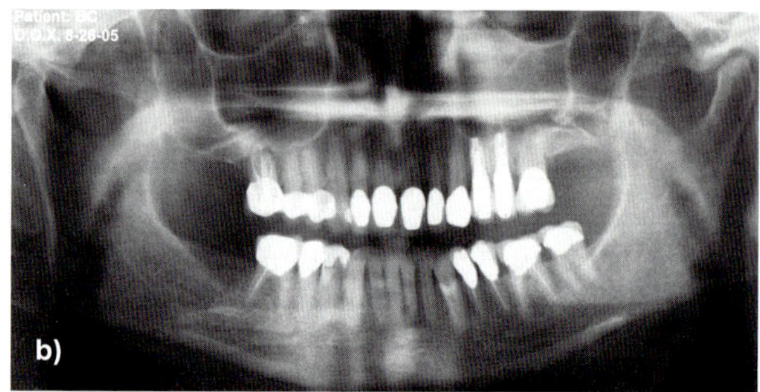

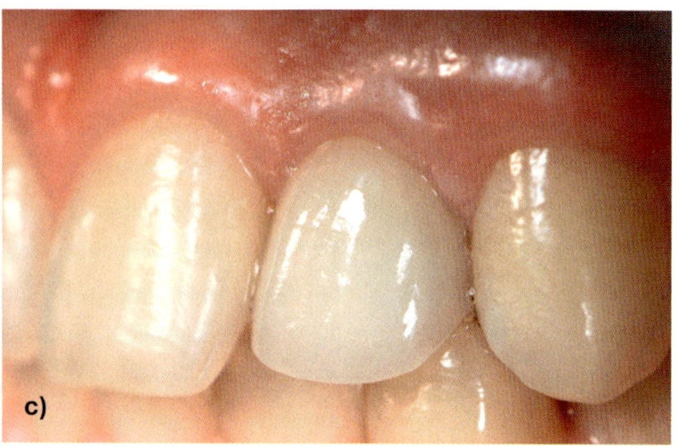

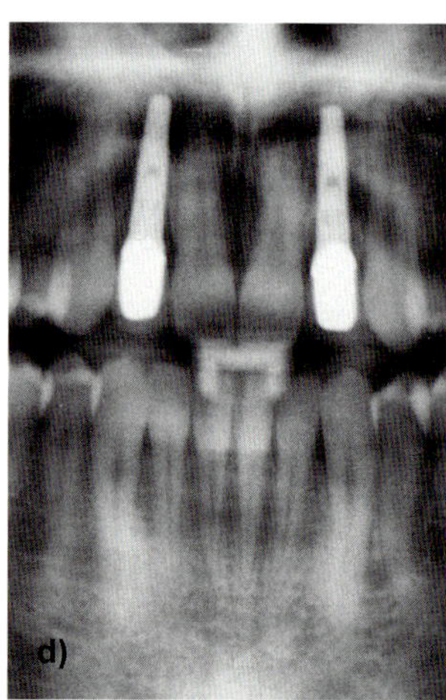

Fig 2-2 **(a)** Partially dentate patient with two maxillary bicuspids replaced with implants. Note the natural contours and interproximal papillae maintained with the implant-supported restorations. **(b)** Stable osseous levels after 2 years in function. **(c)** Single missing tooth situation with the implant replacing the lateral incisor. Note the healthy gingival architecture and contours surrounding the implant restoration, matching that of the adjacent natural dentition. **(d)** Radiograph of patient in Figure 2-2(c), showing stable implants in the maxillary lateral incisor positions after 3 years of loading.

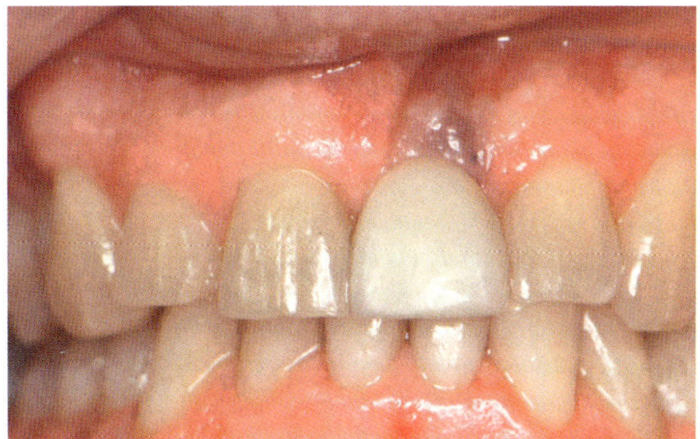

Fig 2-3 Clinical photograph of the failing left central incisor (tooth 9).

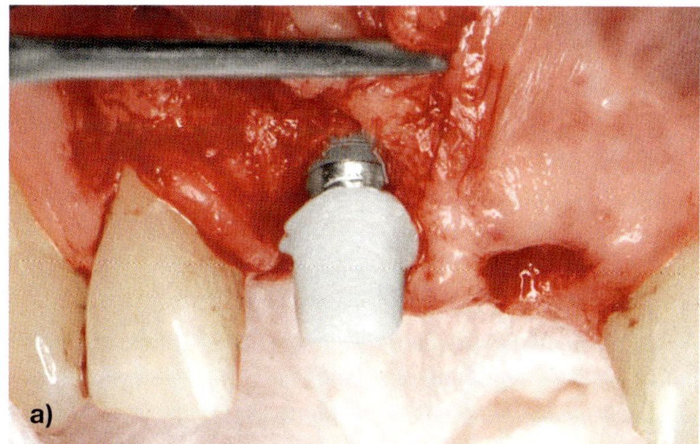

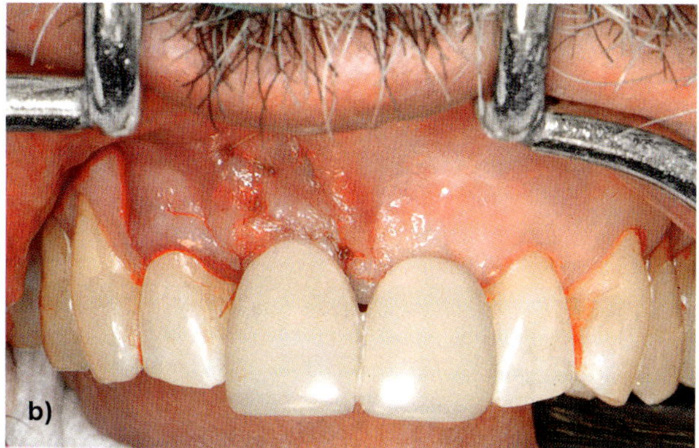

Fig 2-4 **(a)** Custom-fabricated, temporary abutment that has been connected immediately after implant placement. **(b)** Provisional restorations supported by temporary abutments.

traditional treatment protocol. Patients who have fixed restorations requiring a removable prosthesis owing to loss of key abutment teeth are demanding implant-supported restorations that will help them to avoid using a removable denture. This is especially true for patients with a single missing tooth in the esthetic zone that has a failing bonded bridge (Fig 2-3). These patients will not want to wait up to 6 months to have a fixed crown placed into the edentulous space.

To meet the demands for faster treatment times, clinicians have attempted to expose implants earlier and, in some instances, place immediate provisional restorations on an implant that was just placed using temporary components (Fig 2-4). This approach has been successful (Schnitman et al 1990, Balshi et al 1997, Becker et al 2003) but is very time consuming and demanding for the restorative specialist. It also places the implant at risk for losing its initial stability through tightening and loosening of impression copings and prosthetic components on to the implant (Fig 2-5). The NobelGuide™ system was specifically developed to meet these demands placed on the clinician. It gives the practitioner better control of the restorative connection to the implant immediately after placement, and it minimizes the manual manipulation required to deliver the prosthesis by having the restoration fabricated prior to implant placement. Using this system, clinicians can predetermine the ideal location and position of implant(s) based on the demands of the definitive restoration for all clinically edentulous situations (Fig 2-6).

Knowing where the implants will be located after placement with a high degree of accuracy, the laboratory technician can fabricate the definitive restoration (Fig 2-7) prior to implant surgery and have it available for delivery immediately after the implants are placed. Thus the majority of the prosthodontic/laboratory work is completed prior to the

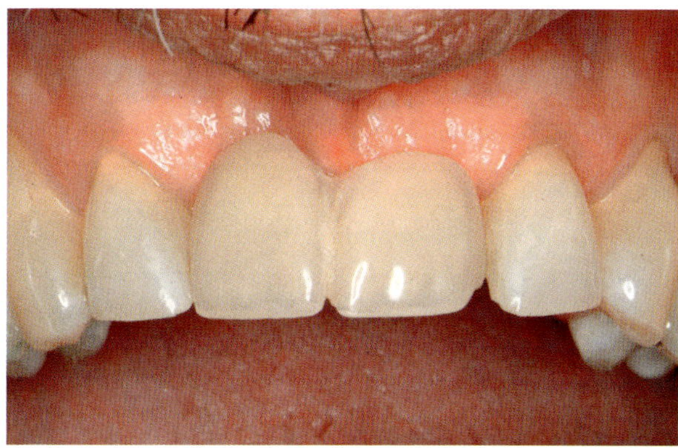

Fig 2-5 Replacing the temporary abutment after contouring the gingival margin of the abutment.

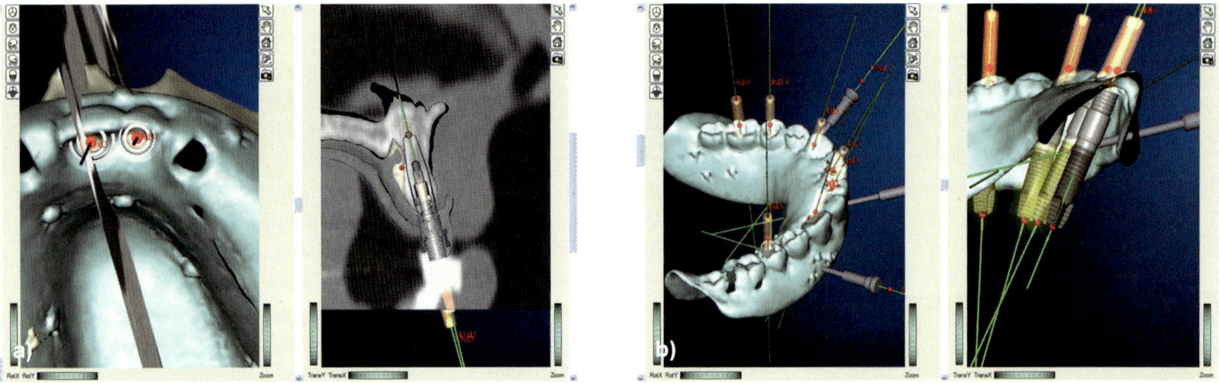

Fig 2-6 **(a)** Contours of the definitive restoration are replicated on the radiographic guide. These will dictate the position and angulation of the implant in this partially dentate patient. **(b)** In the completely edentulous situation, it is important to have the access opening through the cingulum or central fossa of the pontics.

surgical procedure. This saves a significant amount of time for the clinician. The ability to predetermine the positions and angulations of implants is possible by using model-based planning or computer-based planning techniques. The primary goal of either technique is the fabrication of a surgical template (Fig 2-8) that permits the clinician to place the implant into its predetermined position.

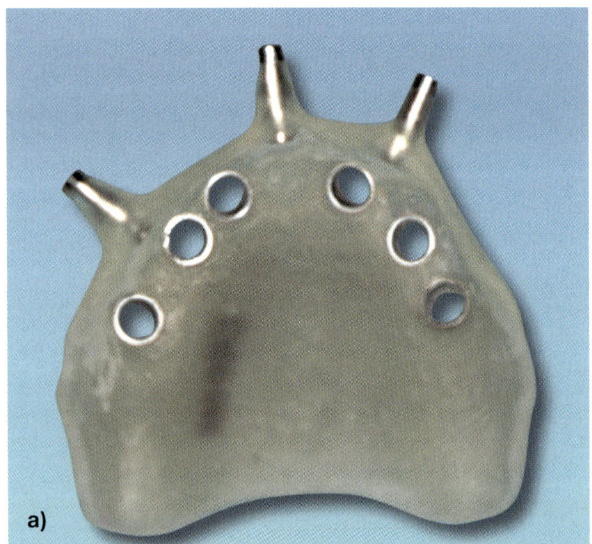

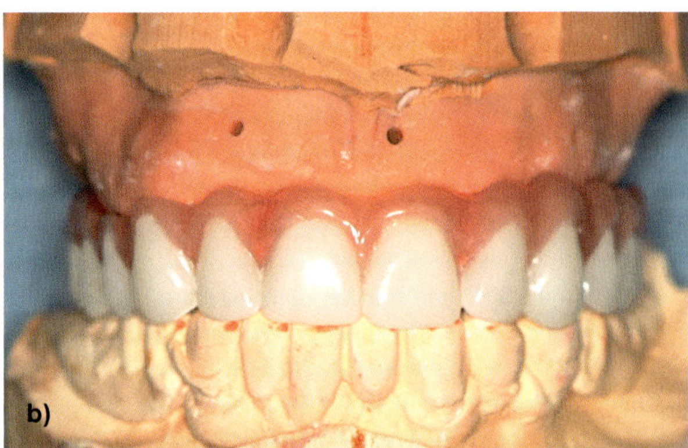

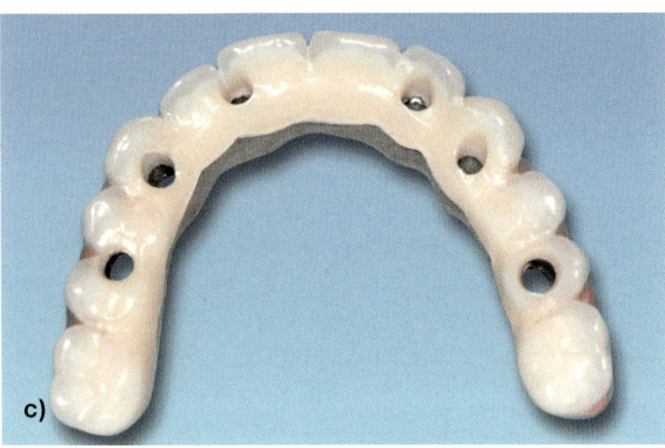

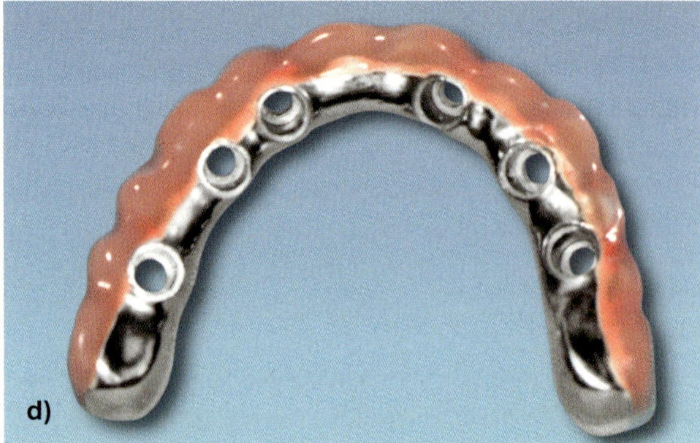

Fig 2-7 **(a)**The surgical template is used to generate the master model. **(b)** Using the master model, the laboratory technician may set up the pontics in the ideal occlusion. **(c)** Occlusal surface of the definitive restoration showing access openings to be in the preferred locations. **(d)** Tissue surface of the Procera titanium frame.

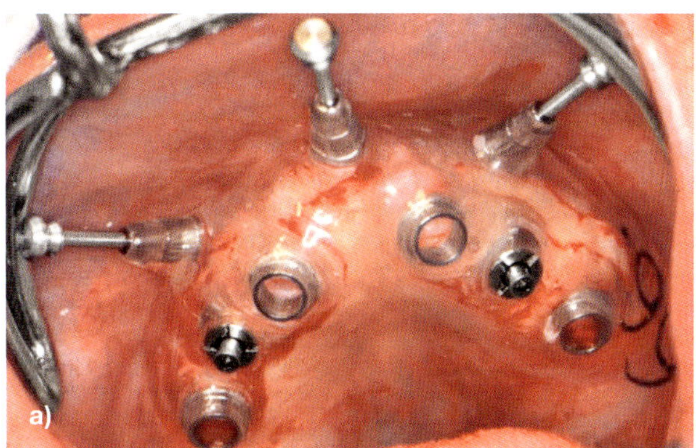

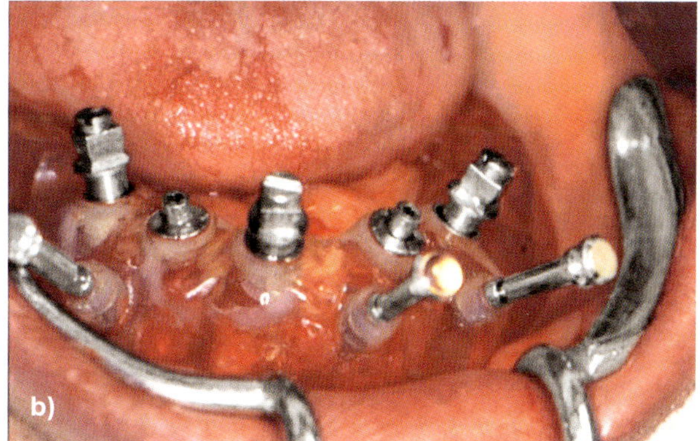

Fig 2-8 **(a)** Maxillary surgical template fixed in position with horizontal anchor pins. **(b)** Mandibular surgical template with all implants placed into predetermined locations.

Prerequisites for successful implants

From early studies on immediate loading (Henry et al 2000, Glauser et al 2001, Olsson et al 2003, Rocci et al 2003), important prerequisites were identified for implants to be successful when placed into immediate function (Ivanoff et al 2001). Achieving initial implant stability, minimizing manual manipulation on the implant that was just placed, and controlling immediate loading forces directed to the implant are several of the requirements identified. Establishing initial stability, one of the most important prerequisites, is achieved through biomechanical interlocking of the implant to the surrounding bone (Fig 2-9); this is necessary to prevent micromotion at the interface during early bone healing. Another factor believed to influence bone healing and implant stability over time is the implant surface characteristics and texture (Fig 2-10a). To optimize the initial biologic response, especially in situations with low bone density, such as the posterior maxilla, a modified implant surface (TiUnite™, Nobel Biocare) has been shown to enhance primary implant stability (Fig 2-10b, c), through its roughened surface, and to achieve secondary stability earlier than machined surfaces through a heightened early bone healing response to the surface (Wennerberg 1996, Larsson 2000, Schüpbach et al 2005).

Another benefit of immediate function is minimization of manual forces placed on the implant during the initial healing period in the first 2 to 4 weeks. This period of time is crucial for early clot formation and the progressive maturation of the clot into osteoid tissue. This critical period is often violated in other immediate loading concepts where the restoration is fabricated after the implant placement. These techniques require the placement and removal of abutments and impression copings, often on the second or third day after implant placement surgery. This important time of

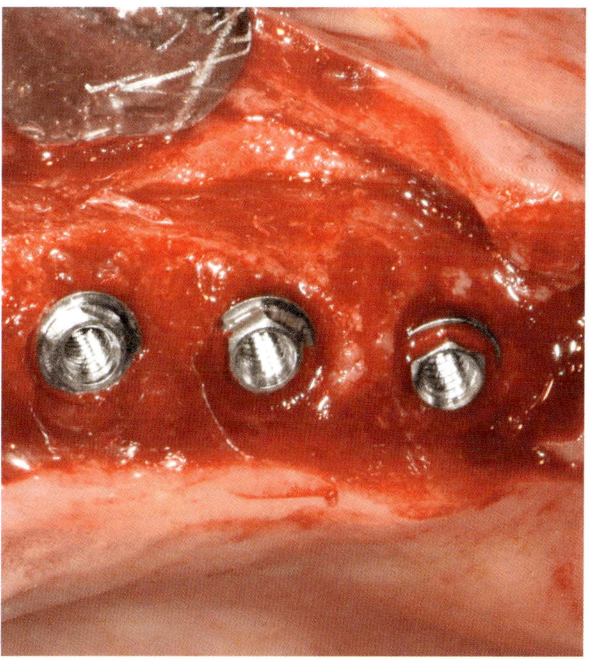

Fig 2-9 Close contact between prepared recipient bone site and threads of the implant.

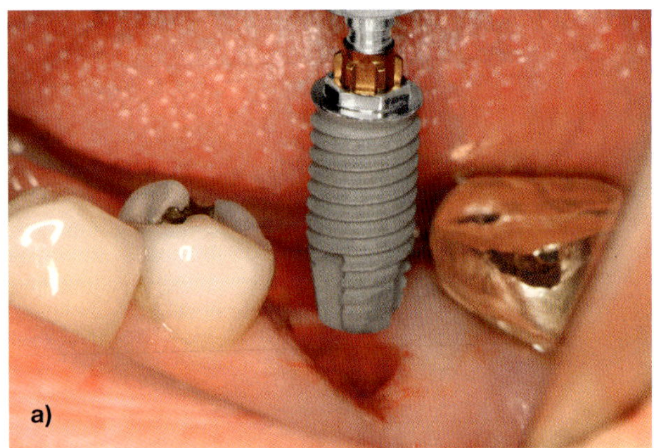

Fig 2-10 **(a)** The roughened TiUnite surface of a Nobel Biocare implant.

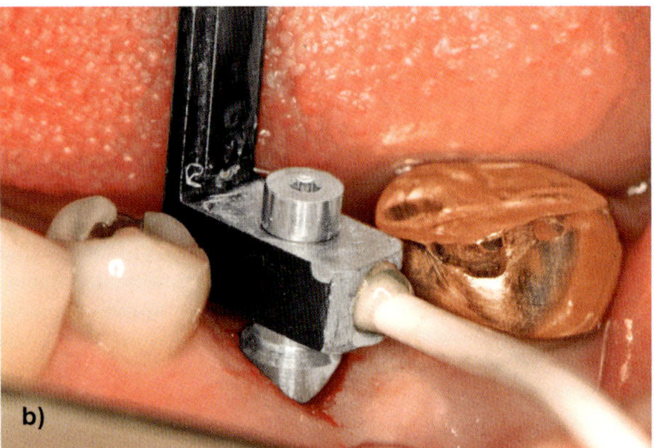

Fig 2-10 **(b)** A transducer from the Osstell unit attached to the implant to measure initial stability.

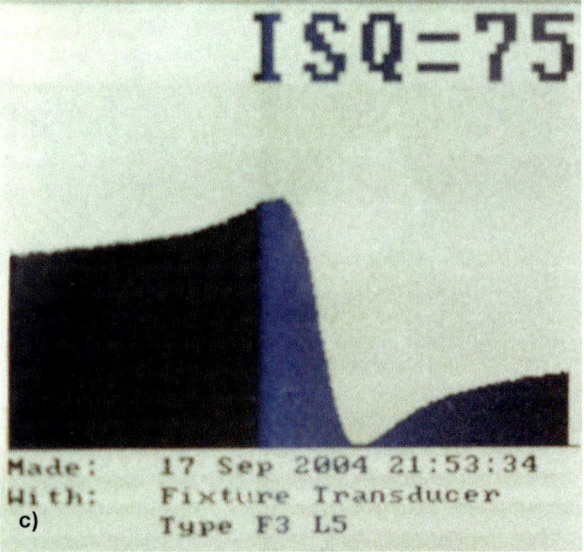

Fig 2-10 **(c)** An implant stability quotient reading from the Osstell unit, indicating excellent stability.

24 to 72 hours after implant placement for the transformation of blood clot to osteoid tissue requires that the clot is left undisturbed and that minimal torque or rotational strain be placed on the implant to avoid movement (Cameron et al 1973, Brunski 1992). This means that any undue handling of implants or components immediately after placement should be eliminated until the bone healing process has matured sufficiently to maintain stability of the implant.

Advantages of the NobelGuide concept

The NobelGuide concept provides the clinician with the ability to control the loading forces applied to the implant and eliminate the highly damaging lateral forces through frequent inspection of the occlusion and contact being made on the restoration. Having the restoration in place immediately after implant placement permits the clinician to check accurately for any contacts during lateral excursive movements and to minimize vertical contact when the patient closes into centric occlusion.

The use of a prefabricated surgical template for guided surgery and a flapless surgical technique greatly reduces the time required for implant surgery, and soft and hard tissue are subjected to minimal trauma, while permitting precise implant placement and achieving a high degree of patient satisfaction by providing the patient with immediate function using a fixed prosthesis (Fig 2-11).

The NobelGuide system differs from other techniques and surgical approaches by conserving both the clinician's and prosthodontist's time and minimizing the chair time required to complete the prosthetic treatment after implant placement. Other immediate loading techniques require the restorative specialist to spend a significant period of time after the implants are placed to provide the patient with the fixed restoration. This may be daunting for the restorative specialist as well as the patient, especially with the time requirements immediately following a surgical procedure to deliver the restorative prosthesis. NobelGuide avoids the need for

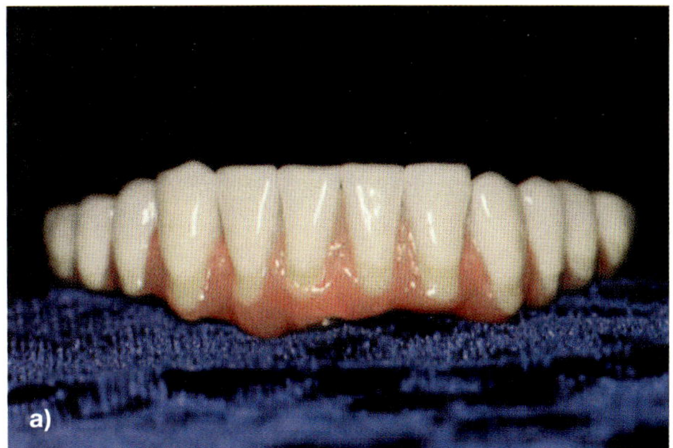

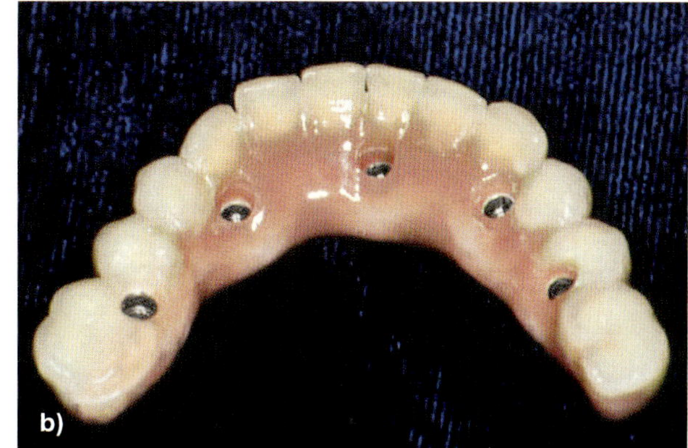

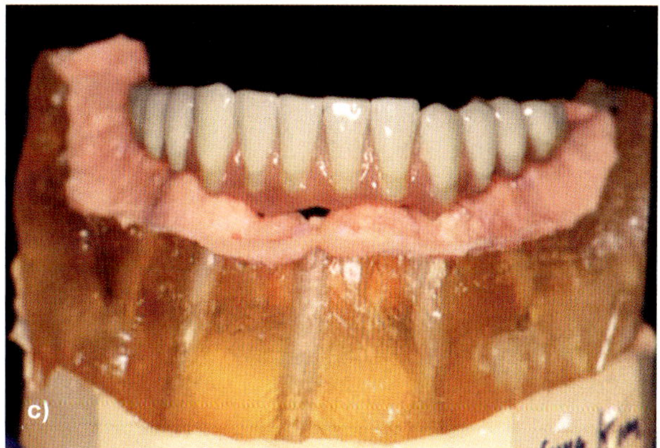

Fig 2-11 **(a)** Facial view of definitive prosthesis made prior to implant surgery. **(b)** Lingual view of definitive prosthesis showing access openings in proper position. **(c)** The definitive prosthesis attached to the master model.

restorative manipulation by having the restoration fabricated prior to the actual placement of implants. The clinician may thus deliver the prosthesis immediately after the implants are placed, rather than having the patient return to the restorative clinician's office immediately after surgery to have the prosthesis fabricated.

Surgical template

The NobelGuide concept was also developed to assist the clinician in placing implants without elevating a surgical flap. The main focus is placed on the fabrication of a very accurate surgical template accounting for the anatomic variations and location of critical anatomy, which will direct the clinician to place implants in the exact pre-planned locations using a minimally invasive surgical technique. There are two methods to create a precise surgical template: a model-based and a computer software planning approach. The two approaches have unique and different requirements but the end result is the same: creation of a surgical template that will guide the clinician to place implants into the desired positions. Following is a brief description of the two methods of planning. For more detailed information on computer-based planning, see Chapter 3.

Model-based planning

An accurate impression is required to fabricate a study model, which will permit placement of implant analogs into the edentulous spaces. The thickness of the gingival tissue over the edentulous site is measured in the patient's mouth using a mapping guide and transferred to the master cast (Fig 2-12). Seven points of measurements are performed: three on the buccal area, three on the lingual–palatal, and one on the mid-crest of the alveolar ridge (Fig 2-13). Measurements are transferred to the sectioned model, where the seven

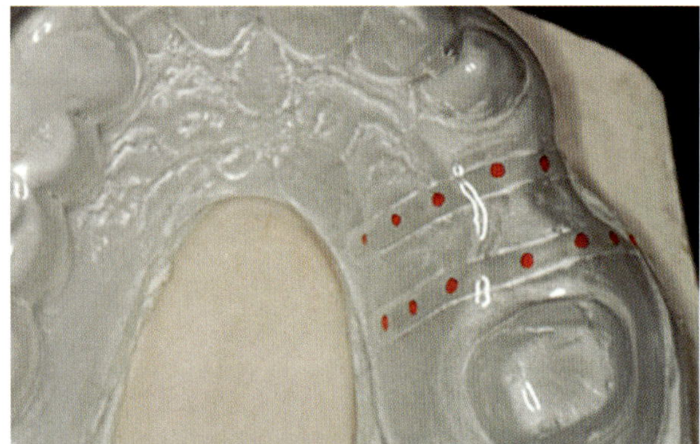

Fig 2-12 A mapping guide fabricated on the master model showing seven sites of measurement: three on buccal area, three on palatal and one mid-crestal site.

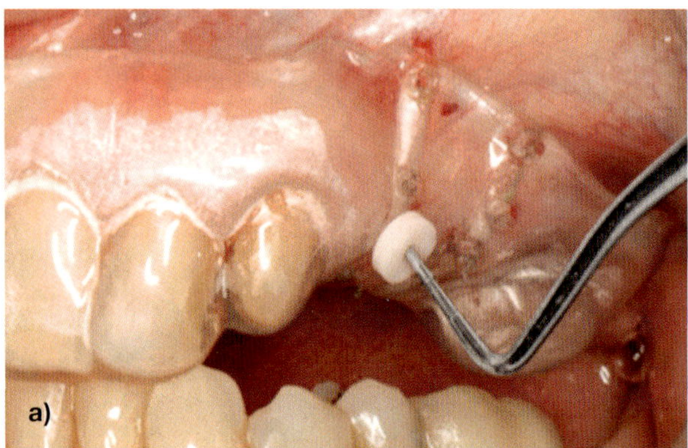

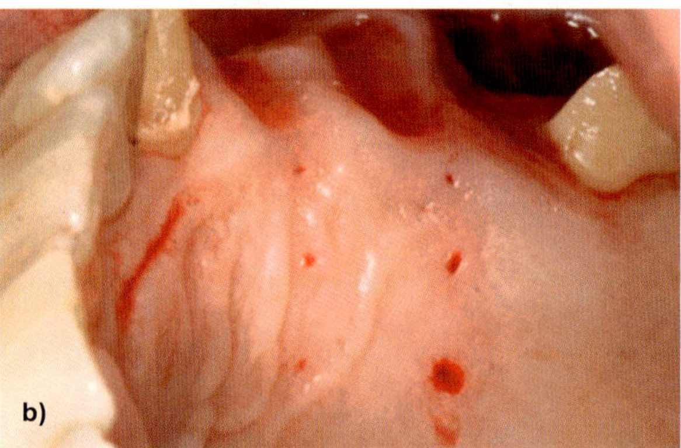

Fig 2-13 (a) Use of a sharp probe placed through the mapping guide to determine the thickness of gingival tissue in one of the three sites on the buccal area. **(b)** Three mapping sites on the palate for two implants.

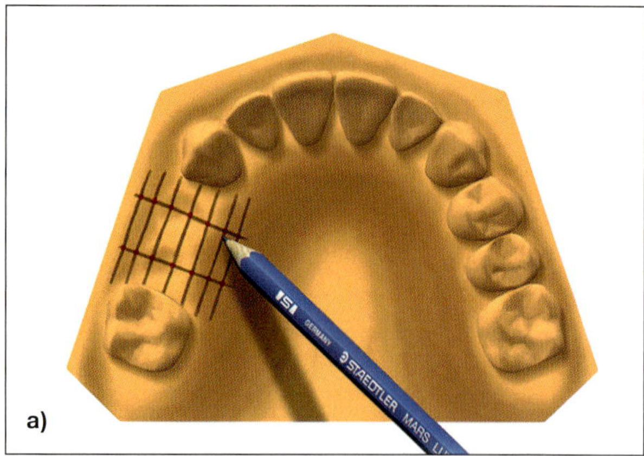

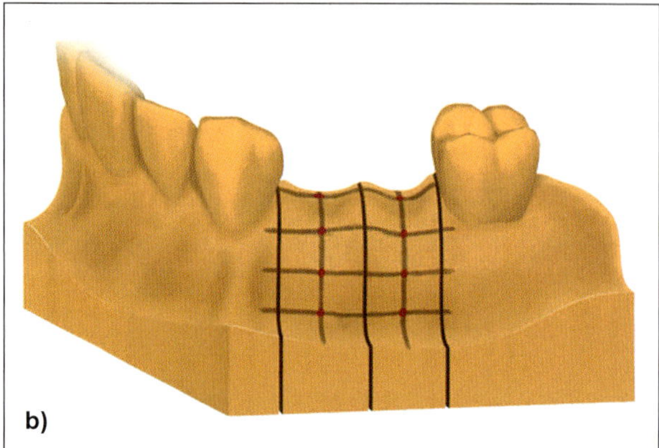

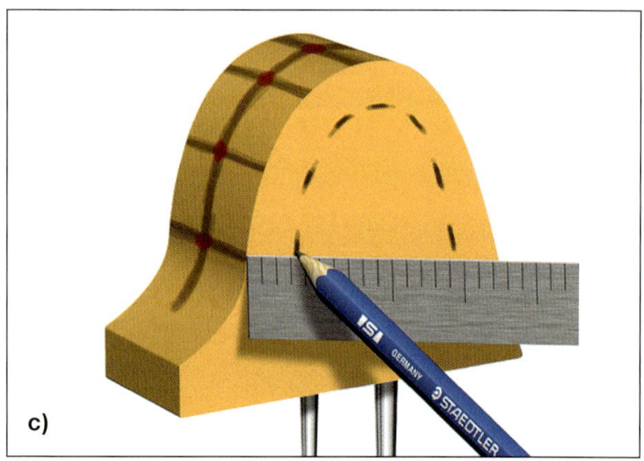

Fig 2-14 (a–c) Seven measurement points per implant site are transferred and marked on master model.

points are connected and the exact thickness of the gingival tissue is removed from the stone model (Fig 2-14). Once the stone is reduced, the indexed segment is replaced back on the base and a gingival tissue mask is poured onto the trimmed model to duplicate the exact condition of the patient's edentulous ridge (Fig 2-15).

Computer-based planning

Computer-based planning requires an accurate radiographic guide, duplicating the dimensions of the definitive prosthesis as closely as possible. This diagnostic approach employs a dual computerized-tomography (CT) technique where the

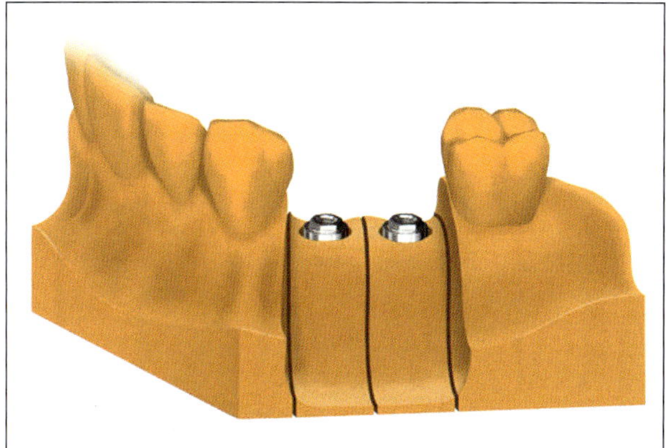

Fig 2-15 Model is trimmed to remove the thickness of stone that mimics the thickness of gingival tissue.

scanned images are taken at half-a-millimetre cuts to create a highly accurate, computerized model of the patient's oral anatomy. The first scan is taken with the patient wearing the radiographic guide with an occlusal index to place the guide in the ideal vertical dimension of occlusion during scanning (Fig 2-16). It is important to establish and maintain the proper vertical dimension of occlusion because the surgical template, which is essentially a duplication of the radiographic guide, generated from the software planning will be seated intra-operatively to this vertical dimension. A proprietary software program, Procera, converts the CT data by superimposing the two scans, aligning the radi-opaque markers so that the prosthesis will be visible over the available osseous anatomy (Fig 2-17). This permits the clinician to plan the appropriate implant position and angulation in the available bone (Fig 2-18).

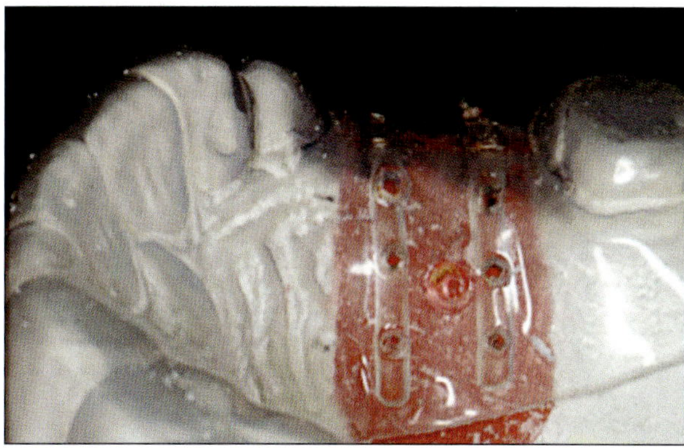

Fig 2-16 Patient is scanned with the radiographic guide and occlusal index in place.

The planned position of implants is captured in a very precise surgical template (Fig 2-19), which is produced from a 'computer-aided design/com-

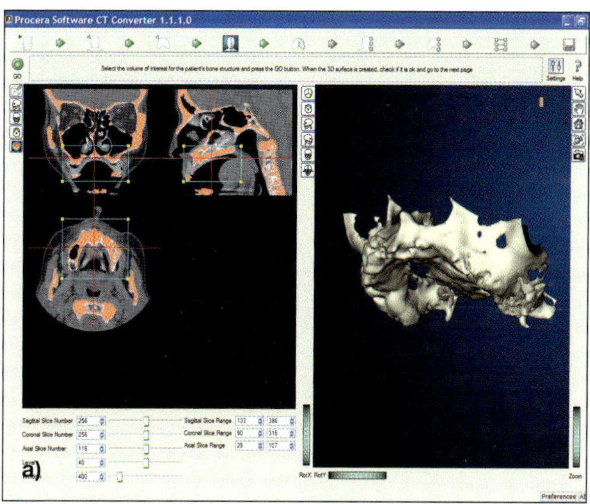

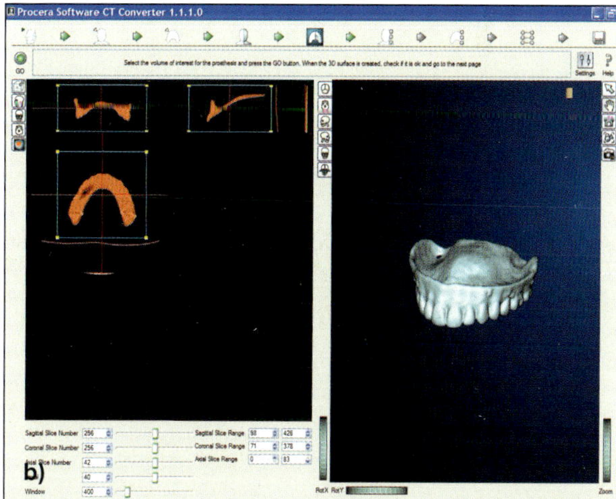

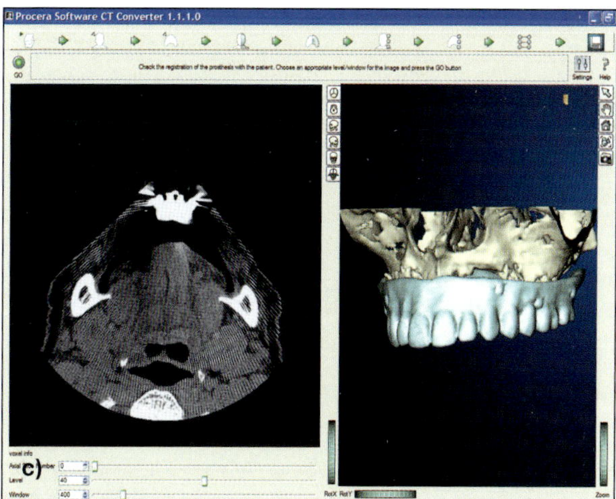

Fig 2-17 (a–c) Procera software planning aligns the radiopaque markers in the radiographic guide and the scan showing the patient's bone structure.

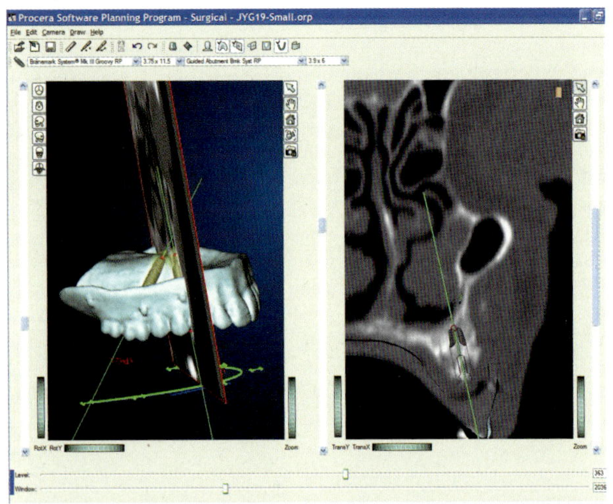

Fig 2-18 Implant is placed into the desired location and, more importantly, into available bone and guided by the prosthesis.

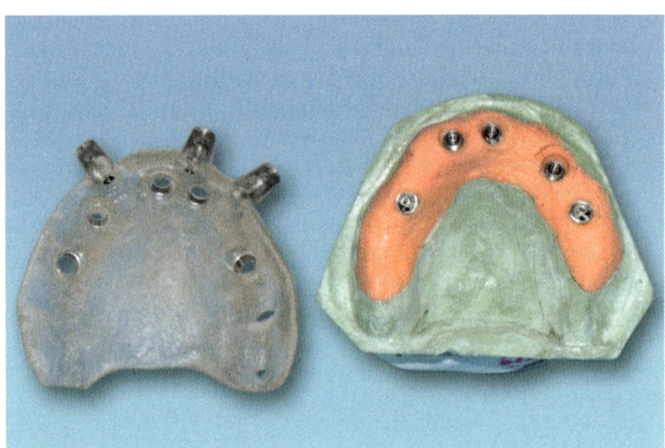

Fig 2-20 Master model with soft tissue cast.

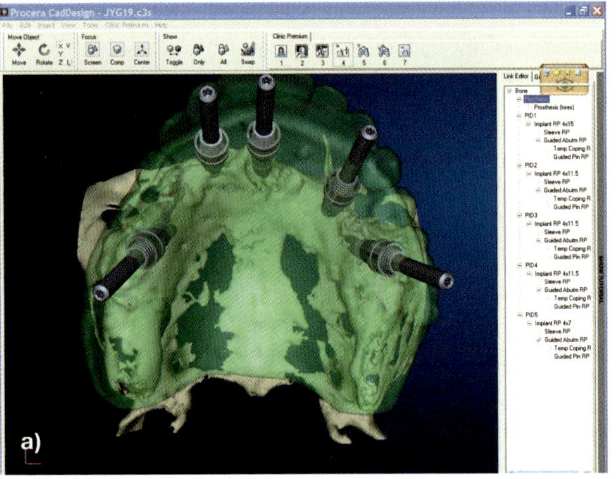

b)

Fig 2-19 (a and b) When all data are inputted into Procera software, a replica of the surgical template is generated.

puter-assisted manufacture' rapid prototyping technique using CT data. Based on the dual scanning of the patient's edentulous jaw and the prosthesis alone (radiographic guide), soft tissue thickness throughout the arch is replicated on the stereolithographic model (Fig 2-20). A soft tissue cast is fabricated to determine the customized height and contours of the restorative framework.

Additional considerations

Other important factors to consider with immediate loading are the fit of the prosthesis to the implant and occlusion. The importance of these two factors is discussed in more detail in Chapter 5. For now, it is important to understand the significance of achieving as passive a fit as possible between the frame of the prosthesis and the implant, as well as minimizing heavy contact in centric occlusion and no contact in lateral excursive movements. Other factors that play a role in the outcome of immediate loading are medical risk factors; occlusal habits, such as bruxism, masticatory strength and skeletal relationship; and gingival tissue health. These factors need to be considered and accounted for to achieve optimal success with immediate loading.

Conclusion

Advantages of the NobelGuide™ system compared with other immediate-loading concepts are:

- reduced surgical time because of the minimally invasive, flapless surgery
- more accurate placement of implants into desired locations using a guided surgical template
- reduced healing time, post-surgical swelling, and discomfort
- minimized risk and complication because of guided surgery and accurate identification of vital structures on CT
- reduced prosthetic chair time and restorative manipulation after implant placement owing to fabrication of the prosthesis prior to the surgical procedure
- immediate esthetics, as the delivered prosthesis is identical to the shade, color and contours of the previously approved restorative setup
- a total and unique system that provides a complete oral reconstructive solution for all clinical situations.

References

Balshi TJ, Wolfinger GJ. Immediate loading of Brånemark implants in edentulous mandibles: a preliminary report. Implant Dent 1997;6:83-88.

Becker W, Becker BE, Huffstetler S. Early functional loading at 5 days from Brånemark implants placed into edentlulous mandibles: a prospective, open-ended, longitudinal study. J Periodontol 2003;74:695-838.

Brånemark P-I, Hansson BO, Adell R et al. Osseointegrated implants in the treatment of the edentulous jaw. Experience from a 10-year period. Scand J Plast Reconstr Surg Suppl 1977;11:16:1-32.

Brunski JE. Biomechanical factors affecting the bone-dental implant interface. Clin Mater 1992;3:153-201.

Cameron H, Pilliar RM, Macnab I. The effect of movement on the bonding of porous metal to bone. J Biomed Mater Res 1973;7:301-311.

Glauser R, Portmann M, Ruhstaller P, Lundgren AK, Hammerle CHF, Gottlow J. Stability measurements of immediately loaded machined and oxidized implants in the posterior maxilla. A comparative clinical study using resonance frequency analysis. Appl Osseointegration Res 2001;2:27-29.

Glauser R, Lundgren AK, Gottlow J, Sennerby L, Portman M, Ruhstaller P. Immediate occlusal loading of Brånemark TiUnite implants placed predominantly in soft bone: 1-year results of a prospective clinical study. Clin Implant Dent Relat Res 2003;5(Suppl 1):47-56.

Henry PJ, Tan AES, Allan BP, Hall J, Johansson C. Removal torque comparison of TiUnite and turned implants in the greyhound dog mandible. Appl Osseointegration Res 2000;1:15-17.

Ivanoff C-J, Widmark G, Johansson C, Wennerberg A. Histological evaluation of bone response to oxidized and turned titanium micro-implants in human jawbone. Int J Oral Maxillofac Implants 2003;18:341-348.

Larsson C. The interface between bone and implants with different surface oxide properties. Appl Osseointegration Res 2000;1:9-14.

Olsson M, Urde G, Andersen JB, Sennerby L. Early loading of maxillary fixed cross-arch dental prostheses supported by six or eight oxidized titanium implants: results after 1 year of loading, case series. Clin Implant Dent Relat Res 2003;5(Suppl 5):81-87.

Rocci A, Martignoni M, Gottlow J. Immediate loading in the maxilla using flapless surgery, implants placed in predetermined positions, and prefabricated provisional restorations: a retrospective 3-year clinical study. Clin Implant Dent Relat Res 2003;5(Suppl 1):29-36.

Schnitman PA, Wohrle PS, Rubenstein JE. Immediate fixed interim prostheses supported by two-stage threaded implants: methodology and results. J Oral Implantol 1990;2:96-105.

Schnitman PA, Wohrle PS, Rubenstein JE, DaSilva JD, Wang N-H. Ten-year results for Brånemark implants immediately loaded with fixed prostheses at implant placement. Int J Oral Maxillofac Implants 1997; 12:495-503.

Schüpbach P, Glauser R, Rocci A, Martignoni M, Sennerby L, Kundgren AK. The human bone-oxidized titanium implant interface: a light microscopic, scanning electron microscopic, black-scatter scanning electron microscopic, and energy-dispersive X-ray study of clinically retrieved dental implants. Clin Impl Dent Rel Res 2005;7(Suppl 1):36-43.

Wennerberg A. On surface roughness and implant incorporation [PhD thesis]. Department of Biomaterials/Handicap Research, Göteborg University, Sweden, 1996.

Chapter 3

Surgical planning

Marcus Dagnelid, Jean Veltcheff

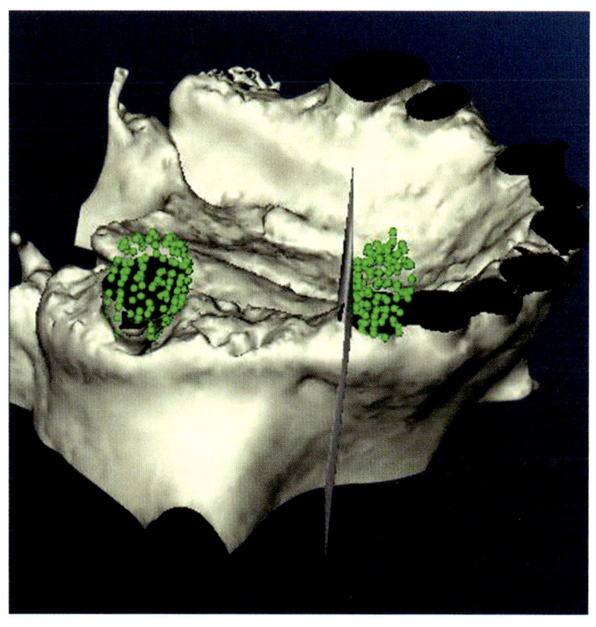

Computer-based surgery at a glance

In the area of implantology great advances have been offered by computerized tomography (CT). Reflecting a mucoperiosteal flap and drilling and placing an implant where there is bone of adequate volume and quality, is still the common surgical procedure. The prosthetic part of the treatment, with considerations for bite forces, height of the bite and lip support, will be based on that surgical result.

With the NobelGuide concept (Verstreken et al 1996, Van Steenberghe et al 2002, 2004, 2005), the clinician can create the optimal prosthetic result; with CT, the clinician can place the implants with the right length and angulations according to the perfect functional and esthetic outcome. CT also gives the clinician highly accurate and detailed information regarding anatomical landmarks, such as the sinus floor, nasal floor and outline of nerves and vessels (Willi 2005).

In modern implantology it is important to analyze and plan every treatment according to each patient's condition. Although the Nobel Guide concept offers a unique opportunity for immediate loading, it should also be seen as a sophisticated diagnostic and planning tool. Working in a three-dimensional (3D) environment enables the clinician to place implants in an optimal position, even in bone with poor quality and quantity, and the clinician can subsequently work with early or delayed loading.

Procera system

Procera software is the tool used when working with Nobel Guide. This software is not only an intelligent system for computer-based surgery, it also includes features relating to the laboratory work, such as designing Procera copings and abutments, and a Procera Implant Bridge.

The software has been designed to make its use as simple and straightforward as possible. By creating a unique toolbar based on seven icons, the computer-based surgery is simplified (Fig 3-1). The clinician can easily access the software at any time and can benefit from surgical planning in a CT-based 3D environment.

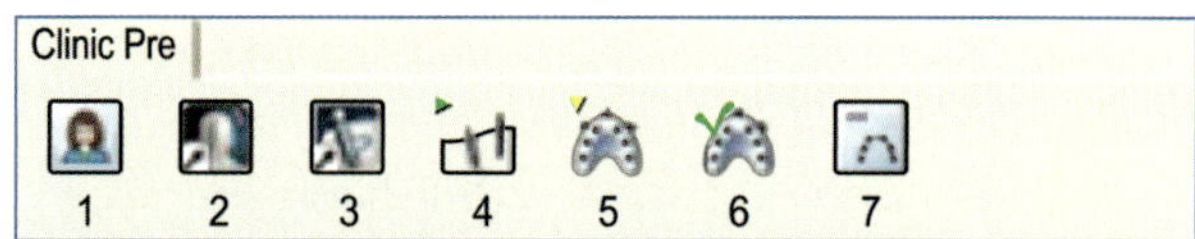

Fig 3-1 Procera software toolbar, which guides the clinician through the seven steps of the NobelGuide concept.

This chapter explores patients' anatomy revealed in new dimensions. It also demonstrates that the use of Procera software for difficult cases assists the clinician in finding the best implant placement. Because of the wide range of possibilities in Procera software, it can be used as a planning tool alone without creating a surgical guide if a traditional protocol is preferred.

Chapters 2 and 6 describe the workflow within the Nobel Guide concept. Before commencing computer-based surgical planning, these fundamentals and prerequisites must be fully understood in order to succeed and have an successful treatment outcome. The pre-planning phase is as important as in any dental treatment, and it is the only way to identify the possible candidate for the NobelGuide concept.

For the purpose of explaining and interpreting the whole Nobel Guide treatment concept, this chapter presents case reports. These will demonstrate the general workflow and also the different tools and functions in the software.

Computer-based workflow

Procera software use begins by identifying the possible candidate for Nobel Guide. Depending on whether the patient is single, partial or fully edentulous, the dentist then prepares the radiographic guide (see Chapter 2). From this point, the clinician will access the Procera software and begin the treatment according to the Nobel Guide concept.

The workflow is based on seven steps represented by icons on the software:

1. register and edit patient information
2. start Procera software CT file converter application
3. open Procera software planning program – surgical planning
4. import planning into Procera computer-aided design (CAD) design
5. create surgical template
6. verify surgical template
7. verify products (drills, instruments, etc.) and print operation specification documents; order surgical template and surgical/laboratory products.

If the clinician's aim is to use the software as a planning tool, the last four steps are excluded.

The radiographic guide can still be manufactured to assist the clinician in placing the implant in strategic positions and in a favorable angulation, although it is not needed.

This aspect will be covered in one of the case reports, where the bone quantity and quality was initially determined to be insufficient and this shifted the treatment into a traditional protocol.

1. Register and edit patient information

Once the radiographic guide is prepared, the patient is registered within the software. This will automatically create an unique treatment identification (ID) number based on a prefix connected to that user and a number for each patient.

All important information, such as date of birth and responsible clinician or prosthodontist, will only be seen by that user. The ID follows the patient throughout the whole treatment and appears on the surgical template at a later stage. Nobel Biocare can easily trace from which clinician a computer planning has been sent.

Most countries have restrictions regarding patient data communicated over the internet. The treatment ID ensures that data transfer adheres to such guidelines.

The ID number created is then used in the printed patient referral to the radiologist. As the concept specifies, the patient will bring to the radiologist the prepared radiographic guide and an occlusal index before undergoing CT with a double-scan technique (Chapter 2). This process is described below.

Double-scan technique

The Nobel Guide concept uses a double-scan technique. This means that two separate scans are made in the radiological examination. (1) The first scan is made of the patient with the radiographic guide and occlusal index in proper position. The guide represents both the missing teeth and soft tissue, while the index ensures the right bite and proper position during the scan. (2) The second scan is made of the guide alone attached to a paper box or a specified foam material.

The density of the patient's soft tissue resembles the radiographic guide; therefore, it is important to have an exact image of the guide outside the patient's mouth.

It is essential that the radiologist has a basic understanding of the concept before undertaking the scanning procedure. CT cannot be properly performed without a correct radiographic guide and index. It is also stated that the radiographic guide must contain a sufficient number of inserted gutta-percha markers working as reference points. The software fuses the two images according to these points, thus giving the true position of the guide in the mouth.

The information generated by CT is composed of two-dimensional axial slices. These are brought to the clinician in DICOM format saved on a CD-disk. To perform the computer-based surgery in a virtual environment, the slices must be converted into 3D models.

2. Procera software CT file converter application

Conversion of the data derived from CT is the second step in the Procera software. An intuitive number of applications will bring the clinician from axial slices into finished 3D models before starting the actual surgical planning (Fig 3-2).

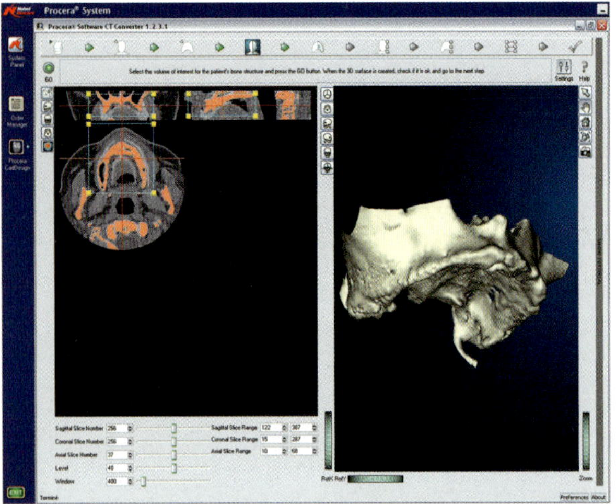

Fig 3-2 With Procera software, the clinician uses a CT-conversion application to change the two-dimensional axial slices into three-dimensional (3D) models. As seen on the right, a 3D model is created from the chosen area of interest in the axial re-slices.

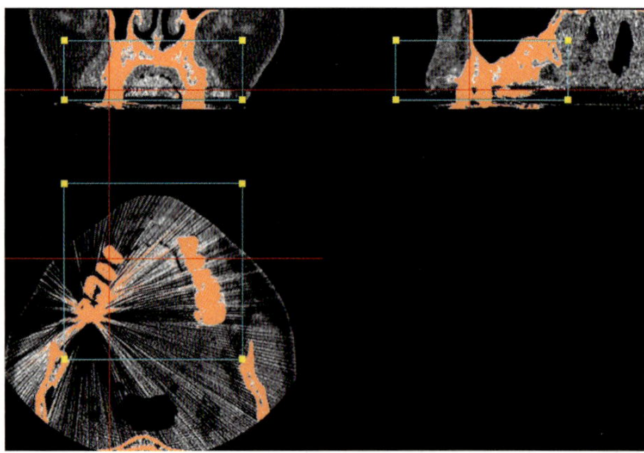

Fig 3-4 In partially dentate patients, metallic objects, such as porcelain-fused-to-metal crowns and fixed partial dentures as well as amalgam fillings, create disturbances in the CT procedure. The clinician can reduce the area of interest and create a three-dimensional model free from artifacts. The original information within the axial re-slices, such as outline of the crowns, will still be available in the surgical planning phase.

As seen in the left part of Fig 3-2, the original information lies within the axial slices of both the patient and the radiographic guide. This original information can be accessed in the entire planning phase and is also the basis for perpendicular, tangential and orthopantomographic slices.

When creating the 3D models of the bone, some parts of the information in the axial slices are not needed for the surgical planning. The area of interest, e.g. the maxilla, can be modified and excluded using the software (Fig 3-3).

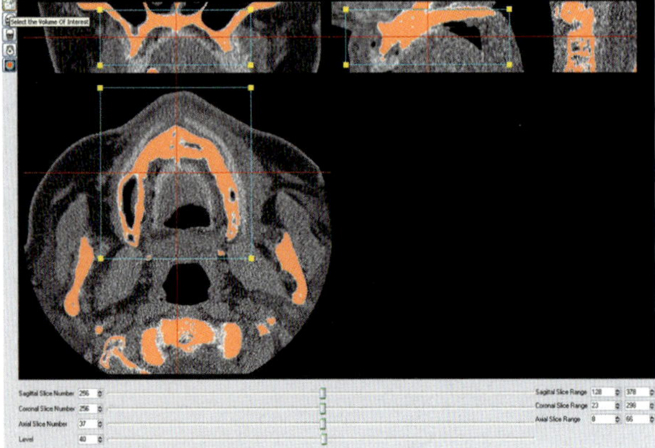

Fig 3-3 Example of how clinician can reduce or enlarge the area of interest, thus creating a three-dimensional model without areas that are not of interest for later surgical planning.

CT conversion is straightforward when working with fully edentulous patients. However, CT of a partially edentulous jaw with metallic objects, such as amalgam filling and porcelain-fused-to-metal (PFM) crowns, can create scatterings. Initially, this can be reduced by placing the patient in the most favorable position during CT, resulting in fewer axial slices passing through objects creating artifacts. It is also possible to reduce the area of interest, thus excluding the crowns of the teeth containing filling etc. (Fig 3-4).

When planning the surgical procedure, the most important information lies in the edentulous area where the implants should be placed, and the root anatomy of neighboring teeth. Although information is excluded in 3D models, the original information in the slices is retained in the system for the clinician to refer to in the surgical planning phase.

After creating optimal 3D models of both the bone and the radiographic guide, Procera software automatically fuses the two scans according to the gutta-percha reference points placed in the radiographic guide (Fig 3-5).

The user is then given a 3D model of both the radiographic guide and the patient's bone, thus providing the opportunity to place the implants in perfect position for the prosthetic work. The dis-

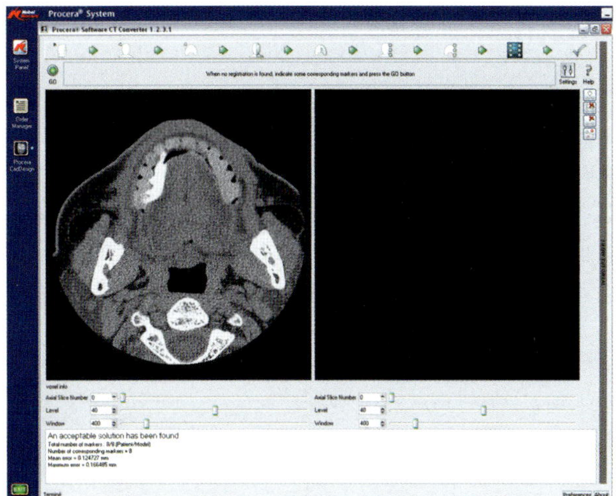

Fig 3-5 Procera software automatically finds the reference points represented by gutta-percha markers, and fuses the two scans according to those points: the fitting is very accurate.

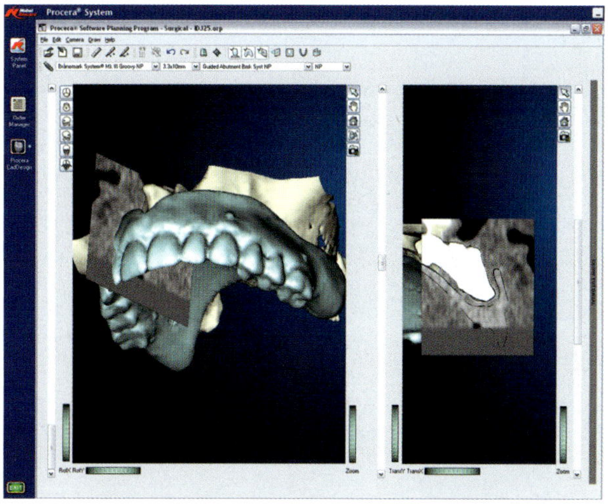

Fig 3-6 Basic outline of surgical planning using Procera software, with a three-dimensional viewer on the left hand side and a slice-viewer on the right hand side.

tance between the two models represents the thickness of the soft tissue or the true position of the radiographic guide in the patient's mouth.

3. Surgical planning

Surgical planning is what makes Procera software a unique treatment tool. Access to the patient's anatomy in all dimensions creates a platform for precise and, in many ways, bone-saving implant surgery.

The user will work with both a 3D viewer and slice viewer simultaneously while placing implants according to most of Nobel Biocare's different implant systems. The slices that are available for the planning are axial, perpendicular, tangential and panoramic. Depending on the patient the clinician is treating virtually, one type of slice can be more useful. This is demonstrated in the case reports below.

General outline

Two different windows guide the clinician in the planning phase. The 3D-viewer enables the clinician to rotate and zoom in on important structures in the maxilla and mandible.

The slice viewer is a window for placing the implant according to the favorable perpendicular re-slice (Fig 3-6).

The software also displays a toolbar, which can be used for showing and hiding objects and other slices, thus giving the clinician a chance to evaluate the surgical planning in all dimensions. Included in the toolbar are features such as measuring distances, angulation of implants and placing points or lines for highlighting important anatomical landmarks. There is also a possibility to visualize abutments, thus guiding the clinician into which one to use in that particular case (Fig 3-7).

Virtual surgery

The implant is placed in the perpendicular re-slice, if possible according to the optimized occlusion and extension of the radiographic guide. The clinician will mimic the drilling sequence and use axes and points to move or angulate the implant.

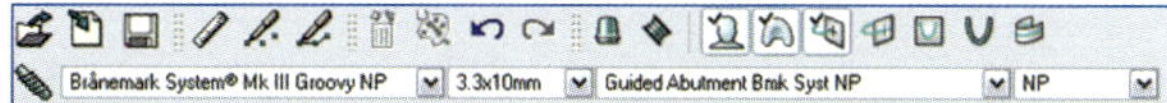

Fig 3-7 Procera software toolbar used during surgical planning. Different slices can be used as well as tools for measuring distances and angulation of implants, and to place lines highlighting important anatomical landmarks.

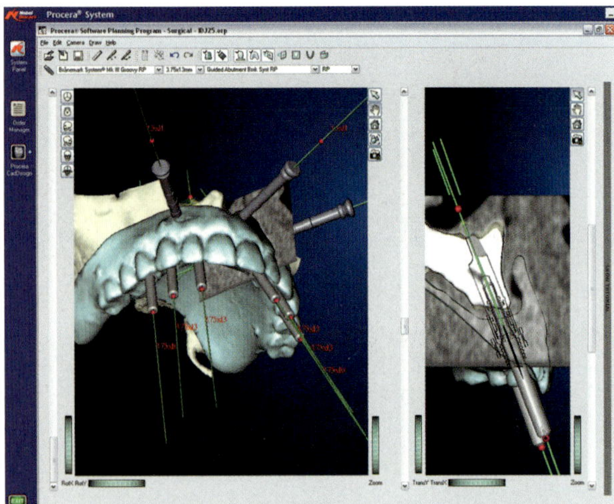

Fig 3-8 Procera software enables the clinician to place implants in a perfect angulation and position according to the radiographic guide. This ensures good positioning according to the supra-construction preferred in the particular case.

In a fully edentulous patient, it is important to place the access holes of the guided abutments in a correct position. The clinician can choose between a screw-retained or cemented supra-construction (Fig 3-8).

As mentioned earlier, it is important to use Procera software as an advanced planning tool in all aspects of implant treatment (Fig 3-9). The use of this type of surgical guide generates a safer and more exact drilling with no wobbling and optimal use of the patient's bone. It is possible to place the implants and then work with common impression techniques at implant or abutment level.

The aim is to place the implants as parallel as possible, simplifying installation of a fixed partial denture. After the installation of an implant, the position according to important structures is easily verified by rotating the 3D model and scrolling thorough different slices. Furthermore, exposure of implant threads on either the buccal or the palatal aspect can be visualized in the same manner.

In the maxilla, the extension of the maxillary sinus, nasal cavity, and incisor canal create borderlines facilitating placement planning for implants. Planning in the mandible is even more defined when it comes to avoiding interference with equally important structures. Several tools within the software can be used to highlight or reveal these structures. Marking the outline of the inferior alveolar canal and its mesial loop is a priority of clinicians; this software more or less eliminates the risks of damaging the nerve vessel bundle (Fig 3-9).

When planning for neighboring teeth in a partially edentulous patient, the software enables the user to mark the outline of the roots and crowns by adding points. As described in the section on CT file conversion (step 2), amalgam fillings and PFM crowns create disturbances in the axial slices. To generate a usable 3D model of the patient, these will be cut away and this, in some cases, will mean excluding information about the crowns of the teeth. The user can still access the original slices and use these for finding the correct outline (Fig 3-10).

If required, bone quality/density can be measured according to Hounsfield units; however, it should be noted that the Hounsfield unit is not a definite value. The clinician should also consider that the values given by performing the general examination of each patient: radiographic evaluation, palpation, grade of bone resorption and general health factors. During surgery, the insertion torque is perhaps the most important value for bone quality. With the advantages of current implant surfaces, and TiUnite in particular, high primary stability can also be achieved even in patients with very soft bone.

Part of the NobelGuide concept is the stabilization of the surgical guide by means of horizontal anchor pins. Depending on the level of edentulism, up to three pins should be placed. This is made in the same simplified manner as for placing implants, but it can only be performed with a proper extension of the radiographic guide in the vestibulum. Placement of anchor pins with penetration to the lingual aspect in the mandible or palatally in the maxilla is absolutely contraindicated. Rupture of arteries in these regions can, in a worst case scenario, create irreversible bleeding and be life threatening for the patient.

In some cases, the amount of bone can be a limitation or contraindication. Advanced resorption with minimal amount and quality of bone can guide the clinician into a traditional procedure with

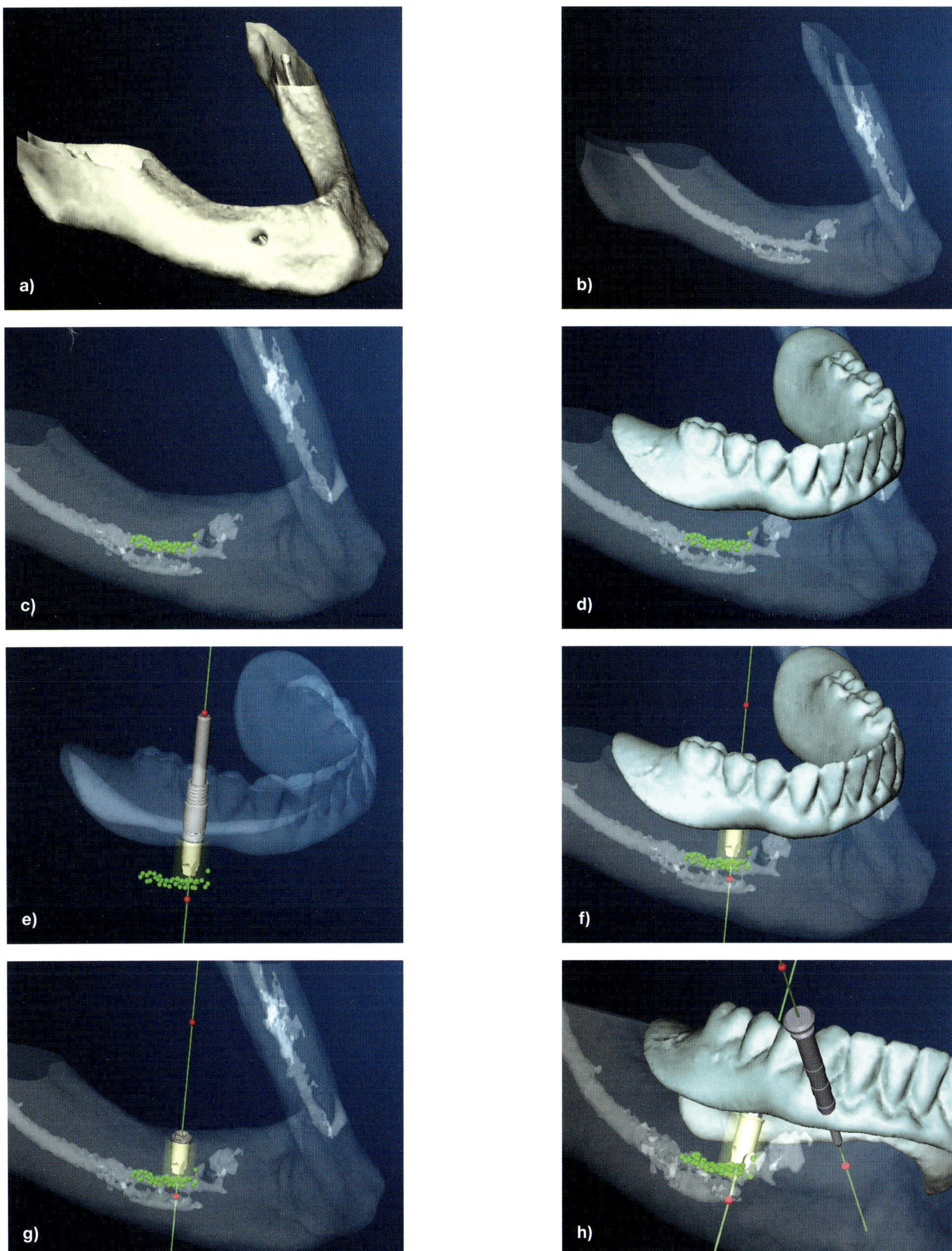

Fig 3-9 (a– h) Different software tools used to highlight important anatomical landmarks. In this case the inferior alveolar canal is visualized both by changing the transparency of the bone and also by marking the outline according to different slices. Together with the surgical template and guided drill stops, this more or less eliminates the risk of damaging the nerve vessel bundle.

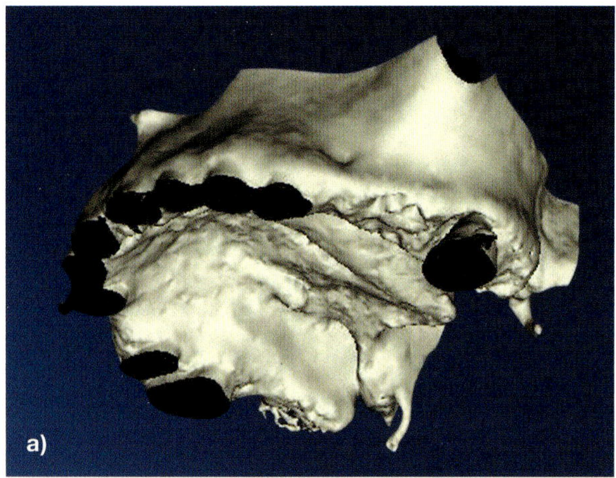

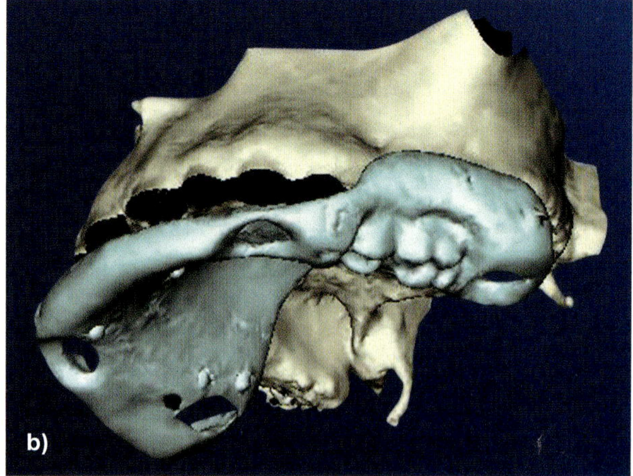

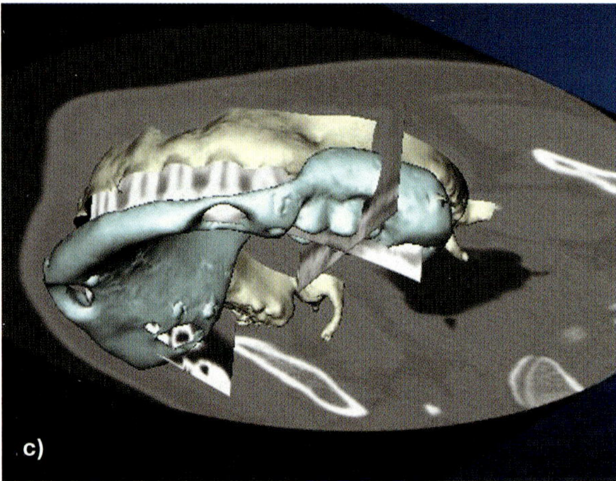

Fig 3-10 (a–c) A partially dentate patient where artifacts created by porcelain-fused-to-metal crowns have been excluded when creating the three-dimensional model of the bone. The clinician can still access the original information in the different slices.

reflection of a flap. Then Procera software can be used as a diagnostic tool revealing the areas where bone can be found.

Case I: female 36 years of age

The patient came to the clinic after many years of absence from dental treatment. She had previously only been treated by means of narcosis and laughing gas, and until recently was receiving medication to treat depression. The patient was willing to begin treatment and replace teeth lost through caries and infections. Radiographs showed problems mainly in the second and third quadrant (Fig 3-11a–c):

- tooth 36 was severely decayed and had apical lesion: the patient also had an extra- and intraoral edema from the infection
- tooth 26 had apical lesions and was also impossible to save owing to extensive caries
- there were some fractured fillings and secondary caries lesions
- periodontal disease was in varies stages, although more than expected for a patient at that age.

Extractions of teeth were made and a removable partial denture was delivered (Fig 3-11d). Periodontal disease was treated at the dental hygienist, and then fillings were performed. Implant-supported restorations were planned in the second and third quadrant.

The patient's subjective request was to replace the teeth lost in the left maxilla for esthetic reasons and economic factors, which made it impossible to begin treatment also in the mandible. Because of

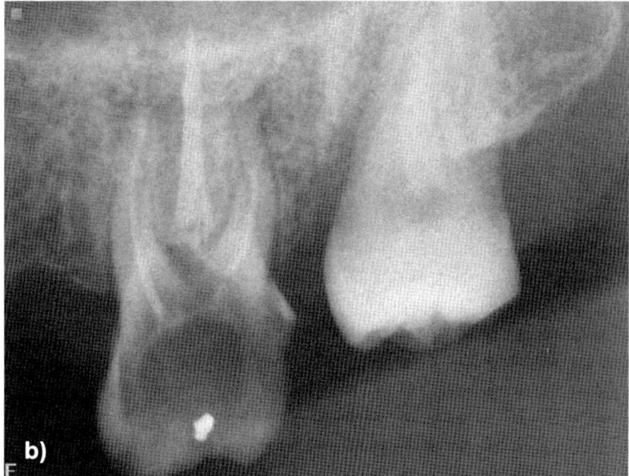

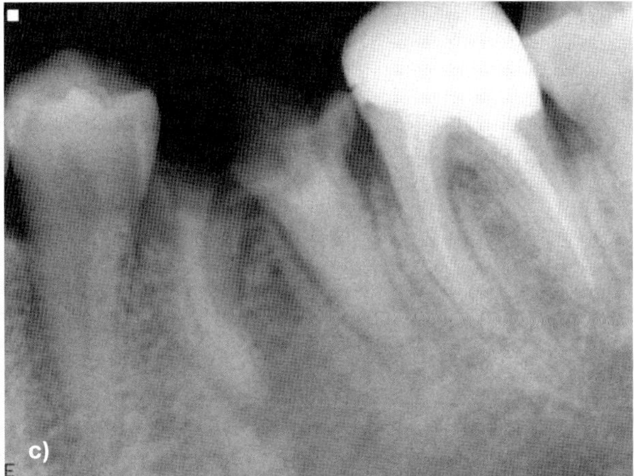

Fig 3-11 (a–c) Preoperative intraoral radiographs indicating a situation with severe caries lesions of teeth 26 and 36, as well as fractured fillings and periodontal problems.

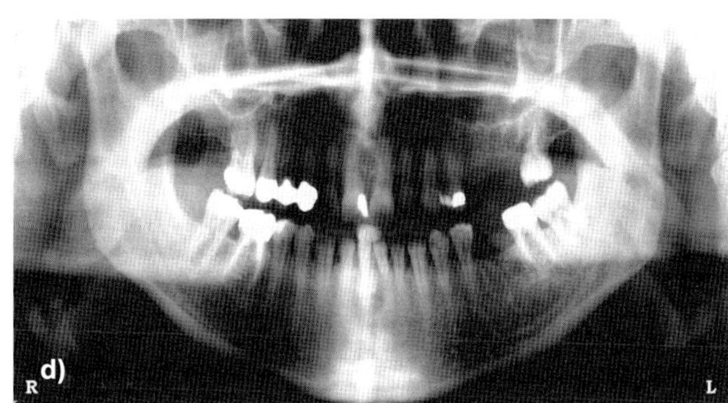

Fig 3-11 (d) Orthopantomogram taken after 6 months of healing.

her previous anxiety and extreme fear of dental treatments, the aim was to minimize the surgical trauma and also the time spent in the chair; therefore, a NobelGuide treatment was planned.

A radiographic guide was manufactured and the following double CT was performed. Using 3D reconstruction in Procera software, it was apparent that good bone volume and quantity were present (see Fig 3-10).

When planning for partially edentulous patients, it is often important to reduce the original information in the axial slices, to exclude disturbances, such as PFM crowns and amalgam fillings. In this particular case, the problem was created by the PFM fixed partial denture in the first quadrant. Despite the reducing factor described in the CT-conversion step, the shape of the crowns and the extension of the roots can be visualized using tools in the Procera software.

The implant should avoid interference with any roots. Also important is the space needed for the surgical guide or, more precisely, the sleeve (Fig 3-11e–g).

In the region of tooth 25, the virtual surgical environment made possible a longer implant than originally thought (Fig 3-11h).

By turning the 3D model and analyzing the perpendicular re-slice, the clinician could see that bone was present lateral to the border of the maxillary sinus. This gave the choice of a tapered implant: NobelReplace Tapered RP 13 mm. The clinician can also verify a bicortical anchorage of the implant in position 26 by looking into the actual sinus region (Fig 3-11i –k).

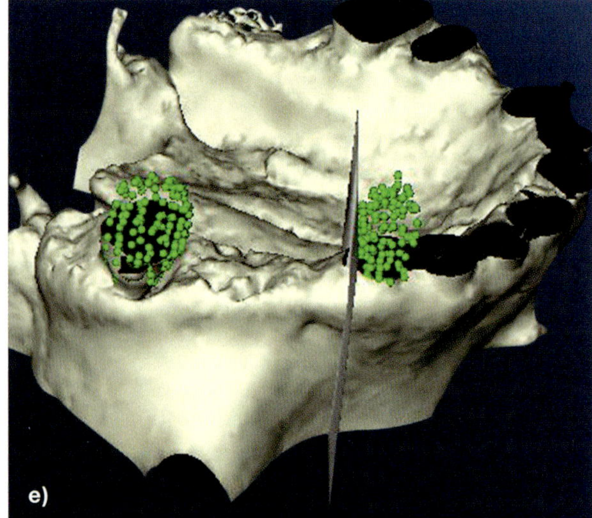

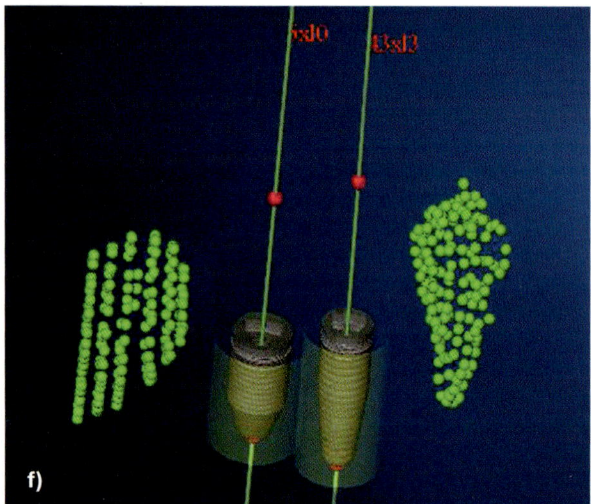

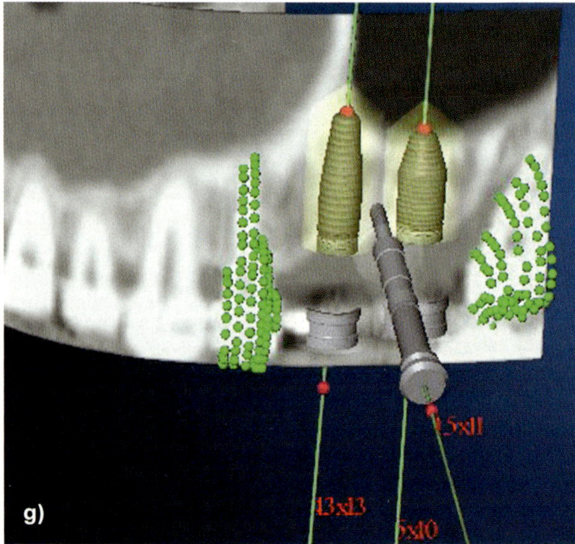

Fig 3-11 (e–g) In Procera software, tools are used to visualize the roots as well as the crowns of neighboring teeth. This ensures safe surgery and that enough space is present for guided sleeves in the surgical template.

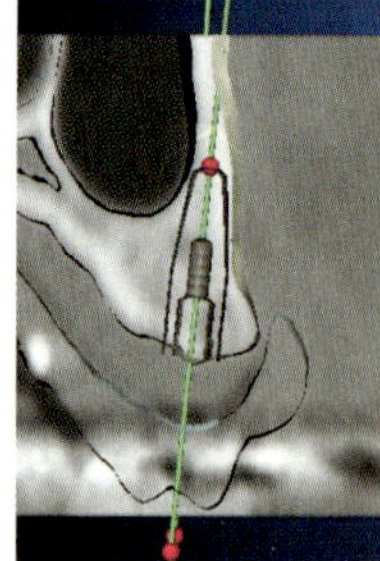

Fig 3-11 (h) By using Procera software and the outline of the radiographic guide, planning resulted in a longer implant than originally thought in position 25. In this case it meant a Nobel-Replace Tapered RP 13 mm implant. Notice also the perfect angulation and position according to the radiographic guide.

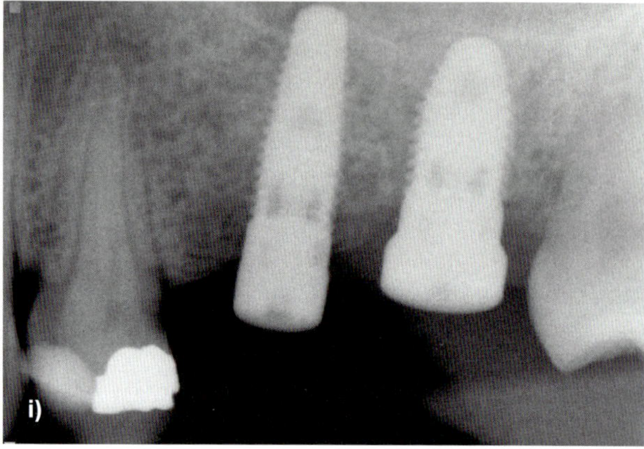

Fig 3-11 (i) Intraoral radiograph postoperative showing optimal positions of implants as planned in the Procera software. Healing abutments were placed and the implants left for a healing period of 3 months.

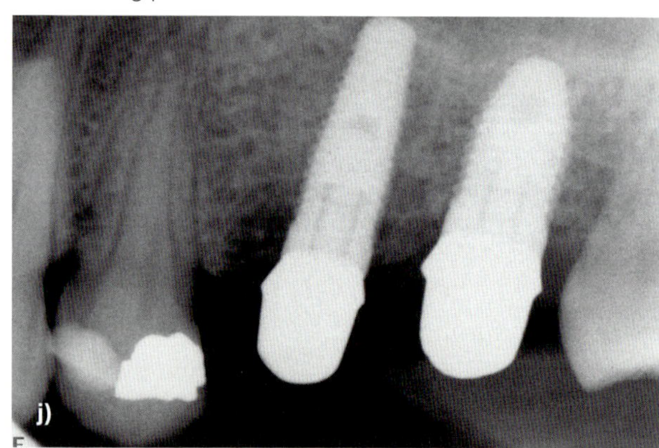

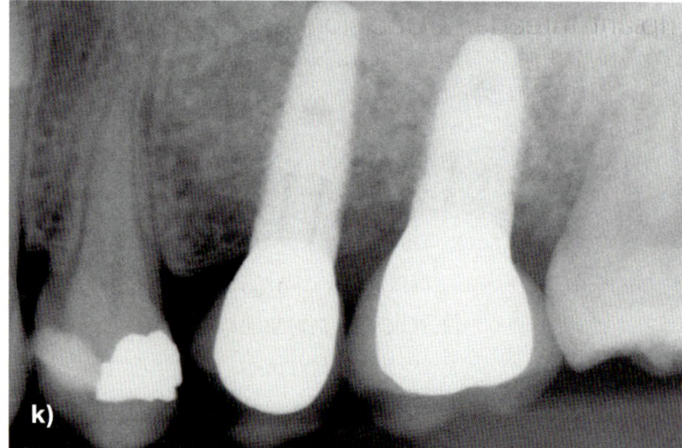

Fig 3-11 (j and k) Intraoral radiographs after 3 months' healing showing the abutment and crown try-in. Two individual Procera zirconia abutments were used with Procera zirconia crowns.

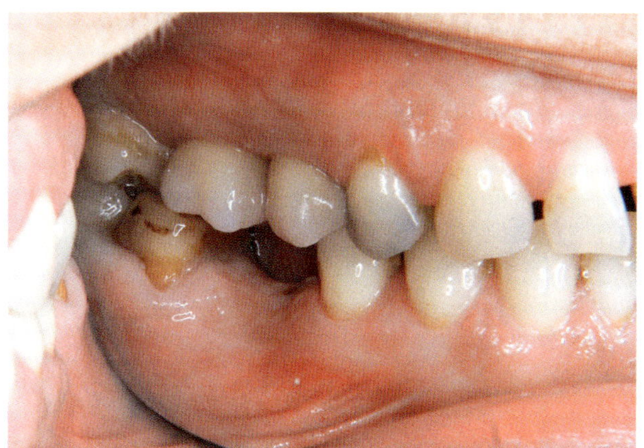

Fig 3-11 (l) Clinical picture of the finished situation. The patient considered that her functional and esthetic demands were fulfilled. Her financial situation did not allow further prosthodontic treatment, and the replacement of 36 and crown treatment of tooth 37 are planned for the future.

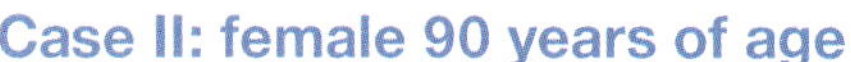

Case II: female 90 years of age

The following patient was referred from another clinician for treatment of edentulism in the maxilla (Fig 3-12). The patient's request was for fixed teeth fast, and an implant-supported fixed partial denture was planned. The first radiological examination indicated a good amount and quality of bone; therefore, a Nobel Guide treatment was planned (Fig 3-12a).

Three-dimensional reconstruction using Procera software showed a very thin bone crest with advanced resorption (Fig 3-12b). Surgical planning was performed and an analysis of which regions were most suitable for implant installation. Because of the difficult anatomy and the degree of exposed implant threads, a decision was taken to use a more conventional treatment with flap reflection (Fig 3-12c).

In this patient, the software was used as a diagnostic and planning tool. The clinician received a lot of information regarding the best implant positions and also where to find bone of good quantity and quality. At the surgical session, photographic records were made after flap reflection. The purpose of this was to compare the correspondence of the situation in the mouth with the 3D models, but also to verify the eventual difference in the final result.

As seen in the figures, the bone is heavily

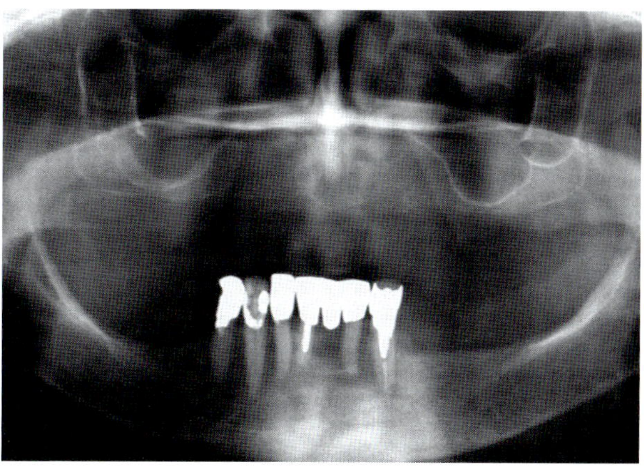

Fig 3-12 (a) Preoperative evaluation indicated what was thought a good amount of bone and quality of the bone in this case.

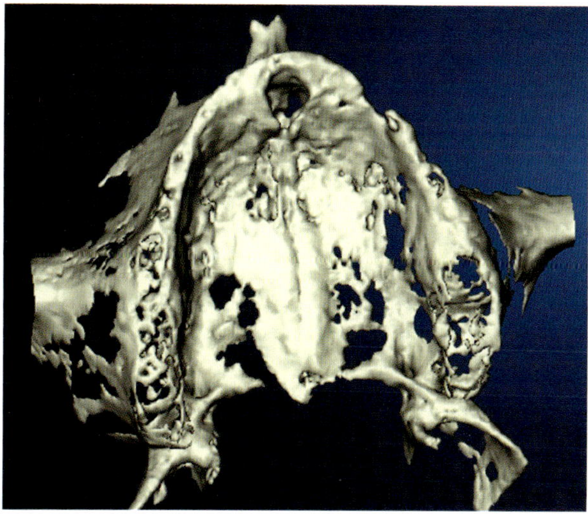

Fig 3-12 (b) In the Procera software, the 3D reconstruction of the bone showed a very thin bone crest with advanced resorption.

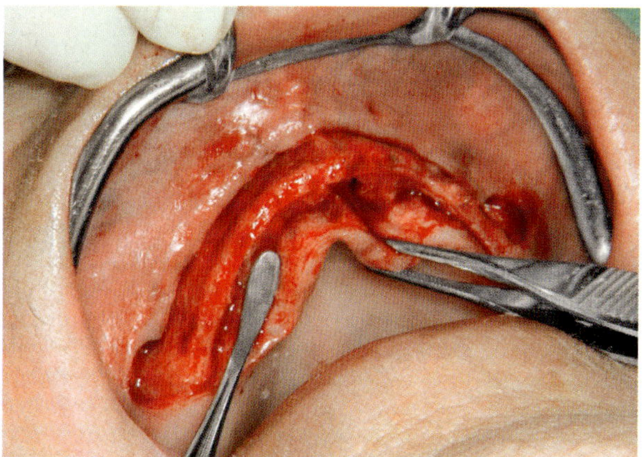

Fig 3-12 (c) After surgical planning in the Procera software, a conventional procedure with flap reflection was performed. This clinical image corresponded with what was seen and analyzed in the software.

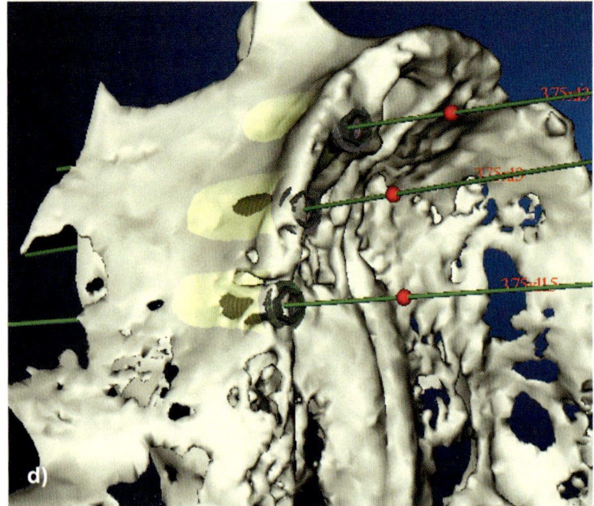

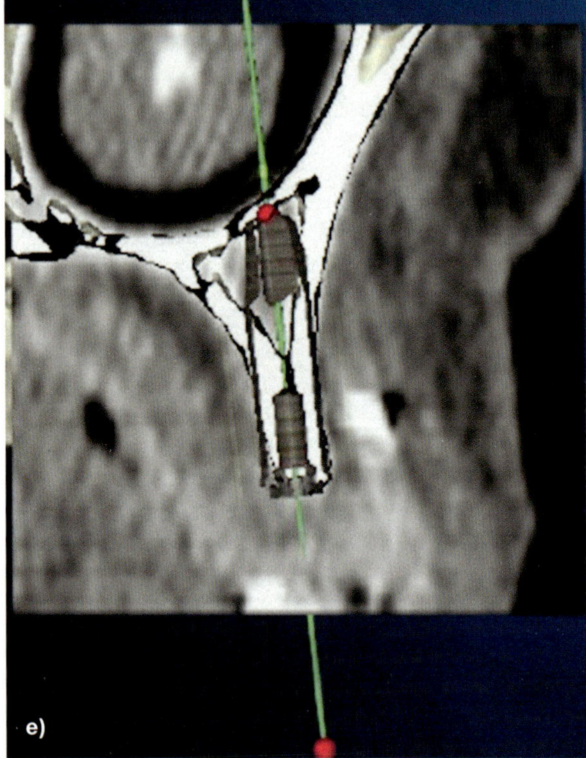

Fig 3-12 (d and e) In surgical planning using Procera software, Brånemark Mk III RP implants were used and the result in **(d)** shows exposure of threads on both buccal and palatal aspects of the alveolar crest.

widened, threads are exposed palatal (Fig 3-12d–g), and implants are visible on the buccal aspect. One of the positions failed and had to be avoided. In this type of case, where primary stability is uncertain and the bone very thin, Procera software can be used for analyzing the patient's bone and for guidance in the surgical planning. Then there is an increased

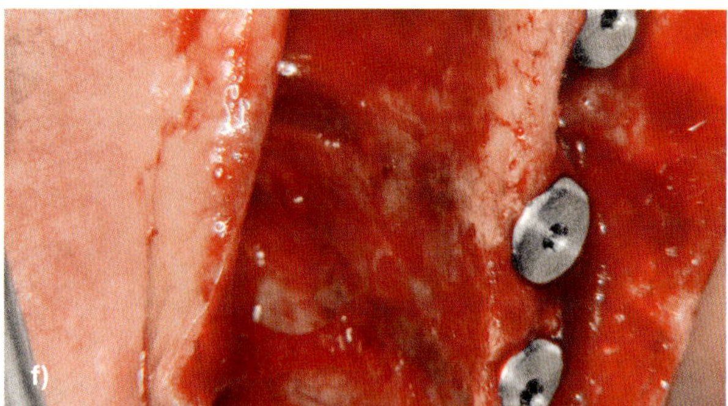

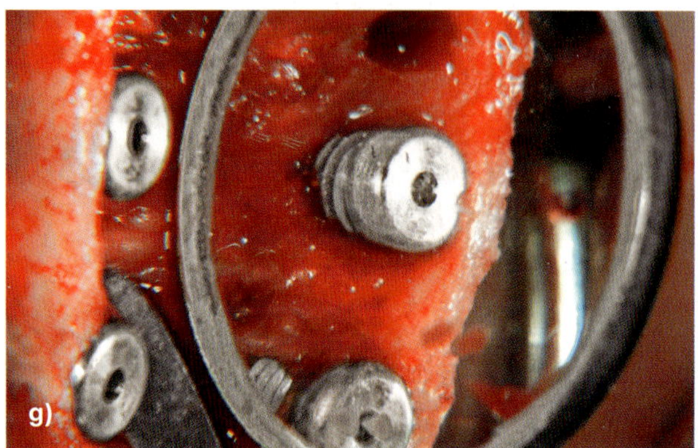

Fig 3-12 (f and g) In the clinical situation, the entire width of the crest has been used and only the periosteum of the bone covers the buccal aspect of the implants. **(g)** Failed implant position: an important factor indicating the correct decision to go for a conventional surgical approach.

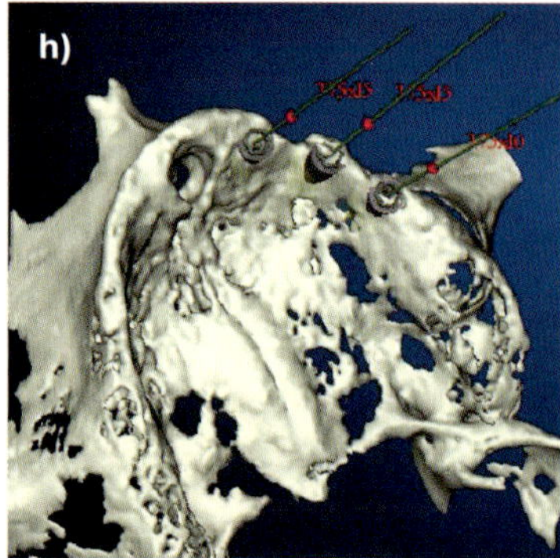

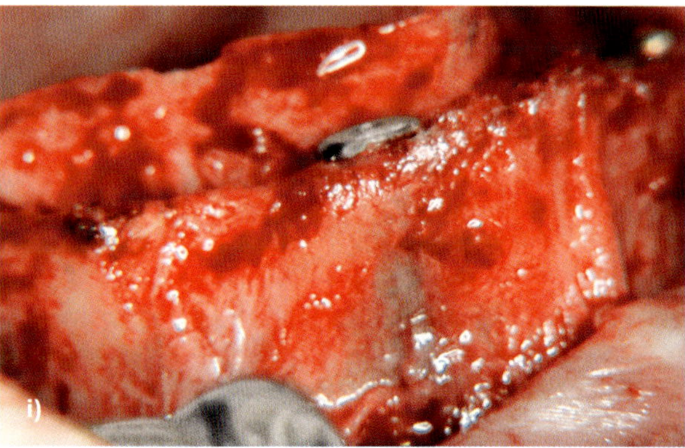

Fig 3-12 (h and i) A similar situation can be seen regarding exposure of threads on the buccal and palatal aspects, both in the Procera software as well as in the clinical situation.

chance of finding optimal positions for implants, and of using the entire height and width of the bone available (Fig 3-12h–i).

Prosthetic considerations

According to the Nobel Guide concept, the prerequisite for successful treatment is proper pretreatment of each patient. Extractions, infections, such as apical lesions, and periodontal defects should be properly healed before sending the patient for CT. Healing must be verified by orthopantomogram or, preferably, by intraoral radiographs.

Grafting procedures or reduction of flabby ridges must be performed in advance. If a radiographic guide is fabricated before bone remodeling and soft tissue healing has occurred, less retention is transferred to the surgical guide. This will also create a false value of soft tissue thickness in Procera software, generating improper implant placement and prosthetic outcome. The clinician must perform an impression for a hard relining by the dental technician.

Surgical planning with regards to the supra-construction is the optimal choice. In screw-retained constructions, an access hole can easily be placed in, for example, the occlusal aspect. If a very angulated position of an implant must be used, the clinician can predict the need of an angulated abutment and thereby shorten the treatment phase and simplify the clinician's communication.

The original concept of Teeth-in-an-Hour from which the Nobel Guide concept originates is, from a prosthetic point of view, the optimal treatment. Controlling the placement of access holes and, most importantly, deciding the esthetic and functional outcome in advance provide enormous gains in esthetics, time, comfort and quality of life for patients. The splinting and stabilization of the implants in a rigid supra-construction make immediate loading possible.

It should be noted that Nobel Guide is an open system: open in the aspect of planning fully edentulous, partial, or single cases. The supra-construction can be provisional or final, screw retained or cemented. The possibility remains to place healing abutments after the flapless surgery and work with impressions on implant or abutment level.

Interactive communication

In all kinds of treatment, proper information is the key to a successful treatment outcome. Also in cases where a patient is expressing hesitation, detailed information about a specific procedure can overcome insecurity and anxiety in the patient.

Procera software in itself can be used as a tool to include the patient in the planning phase. The clinician can easily show the patient the flow of the concept with computer-based planning. Snapshots can be taken as well as movie clips in the planning phase, serving as material for communication.

In modern dentistry, the aim is also to develop and widen the communication between the clinician and dental technician. Different versions of Procera software can be used, sharing planning files and creating a forum for both surgical and prosthetic discussions. The esthetic and functional outcome is a direct result of this close collaboration.

The communication between the prosthodontist and clinician is also an important factor for a successful treatment outcome. Again, both parties can access the planning via similar versions of the Procera software, discussing possible implant positions and angulations, and the influence these will have on the prosthetic treatment.

4. Import planning into Procera CAD

Completed surgical planning is saved in a designated folder for each patient. This planning will be imported to the computer-aided design (CAD) system and will provide an initial outline of the surgical template.

5. Create surgical template

This step will generate the finished surgical template. If there is an error within the surgical planning, e.g. collision between implants, implants and anchor pins, or interference with the supra-construction, the clinician can return to surgical planning (step 3) in the software. In the surgical planning step, the required change can be made; steps 4 and 5 will generate the proper outline of the new surgical template.

6. Verify surgical template

The computer will automatically verify the planning and surgical template. If there still is an error, the clinician will be forced to return to step 3 once more.

It should be pointed out that there is no system included that warns the clinician of interference with anatomical landmarks. The responsibility rests on the clinician's proper knowledge of each patient's anatomy.

7. Verify products

In the last step of the Procera software, the computer will automatically calculate products needed according to the surgical planning. If Brånemark System implants are used, the drills are single use, compared with, for example, Replace Systems' multiple use of drills.

The clinician can add or withdraw any products in the Nobel Biocare portfolio. Once the order list is prepared, an order is sent to Nobel Biocare and the products are delivered within 10 days worldwide.

The surgical guide is manufactured by Nobel Biocare and this is brought in a separate package.

From this point forward, the dental technician will use the surgical guide to manufacture a stone model from which the prosthetic work is manufactured. The unique treatment ID for each patient will be seen on all products, thus simplifying communication between everyone involved in the treatment.

The clinician can also have a printout with a schematic drawing of the surgical planning together with the list of products to be used. This can be helpful, for example when using implants of different lengths in different positions, to avoid overpreparation and potential risks of interference with vital structures.

Particularly in the mandible, the clinician must rely on measurements made in the software and use the guided drill stops according to each implant length.

Conclusion

In the age of computer technology and 3D environments in particular, the field of implant dentistry will gradually change from a traditional planning protocol into a computerized one. More implant surgery will occur as a flapless procedure, minimizing the surgical trauma and improving patients' comfort. A successful treatment outcome can in many ways be foreseen.

The use of CT for surgical planning is not a new concept. But the assembly of all the benefits generated by that technology into a highly simplified, exact and user-friendly tool is, in the authors' opinion, available for the first time in the Nobel Guide concept.

As this concept develops along with the technology, clinicians will have access to safer and more precise treatment alternatives and, most importantly, will be able to offer significant patient benefits. After all, the main focus is the patient and improving quality of life for those with various stages of edentulism.

References

van Steenberghe D, Naert D, Andersson M, Brajnovic I, Van Cleynenbreugel J, Seutens P. A custom template and definitive prosthesis allowing immediate implant loading in the maxilla: a clinical report. Int J Oral Maxillofac Implants 2002;17:663-670.

van Steenberghe D, Ericsson I, Van Cleynenbreugel J, Schutser F, Brajnovic I, Andersson M. High precision planning for oral implants based on 3D CT scanning. A new surgical technique for immediate and delayed loading. Appl Osseointegration Res 2004;4:27-31.

van Steenberghe D, Glauser R, Blombäck U, Andersson M, Schutyser F, Pettersson A & Wendelhag I. A computed tomographic scan-derived customized surgical template and fixed prosthesis for flapless surgery and immediate loading of implants in fully edentulous maxillae: a prospective multicenter study. Clin Implant Dent Relat Res 2005:7:S111-120.

Verstreken K, Van Cleynenbreugel J, Marcahl G, Naert I, Suetens P, Van Steenberghe D. Computer-assisted planning of oral implant surgery: a three-dimensional approach. Int J Oral Maxillofac Implants 1996:11:806-810.

Willi A. Kalender computed tomography: fundamentals, system technology, image quality, applications (2nd ed). Publicis Corporate Publishing, 2005.

Chapter 4

NobelGuide in use

Part I: NobelGuide surgery

Peter K Moy, Patrick Palacci

Part II: NobelGuide, zygoma implants and immediate function

Chantal Malevez

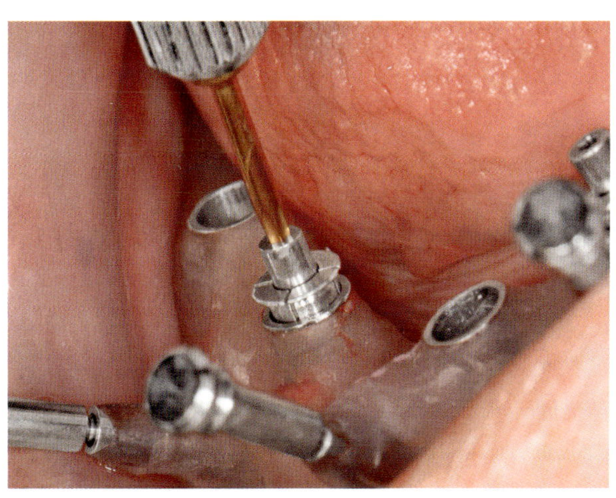

Part I: NobelGuide surgery

Since the introduction of Teeth-in-an-Hour in 2003 for the completely edentulous patient, the technique has evolved into one that can be used for any clinical situation: the completely edentulous patient (Horiuchi et al 2000), the partially dentate (Glauser et al 2001) and the single-missing tooth (Ericsson et al 2001). Each edentulous situation requires slight modifications in the pre-surgical workup and in the surgical approach. The specific diagnostic workup for each of the three varieties of edentulism is discussed in detail in Chapter 6.

This chapter outlines the surgical technique for each state of edentulism. The procedure is described for the completely edentulous patient, then variations in surgical technique used for patients who are partially dentate and have a single-missing tooth are discussed.

Surgical procedure

When using the NobelGuide technique, the sequence of twist drills and surgical components is the same for all edentulous clinical situations. When the surgical template is returned from the laboratory, the first thing that the clinician should do is perform a general inspection to ensure that the identification number on the template matches that of the planning identification number assigned to that patient. The clinician should check that the configuration of the guide sleeves and planned number of implants in the surgical template are identical to the operation information sheet from the planning software (Figs 4-1 and 4-2). The template should also be inspected to ensure there is no warping or damage to the acrylic or guide sleeves within the template.

The clinician should connect the laboratory-fabricated surgical occlusal index to the surgical template and ensure that the fit is exact. The surgical index must also have a tight fit to the dentition in the opposing dental arch (Fig 4-3). The precise fit of the surgical occlusal index ensures that the surgical template will be secured to the dental arch in the proper vertical dimension of occlusion (Fig 4-4). If the surgical template is not placed at the proper vertical dimension during the surgery, the implants placed through the template will not be seated to the proper vertical position within the alveolar ridge, and the fixed partial denture that will be connected after implant placement will either be in infra- or hyper-occlusion.

The surgical procedure is started by administering local anesthetic, with care to avoid excessive displacement of the gingival tissue, thus

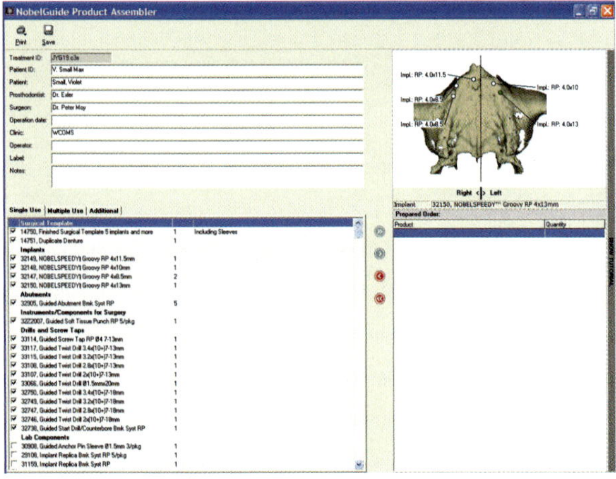

Fig 4-1 (a) Order sheet from NobelGuide planning program with the patient's treatment identification number.

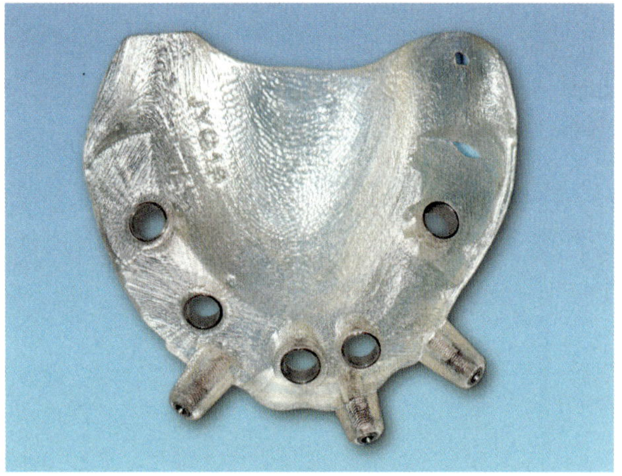

Fig 4-1 (b) Surgical template with patient's treatment identification number (upper left corner) is typically placed by the palatal vault of the maxillary template and the lingual flange of the mandibular template.

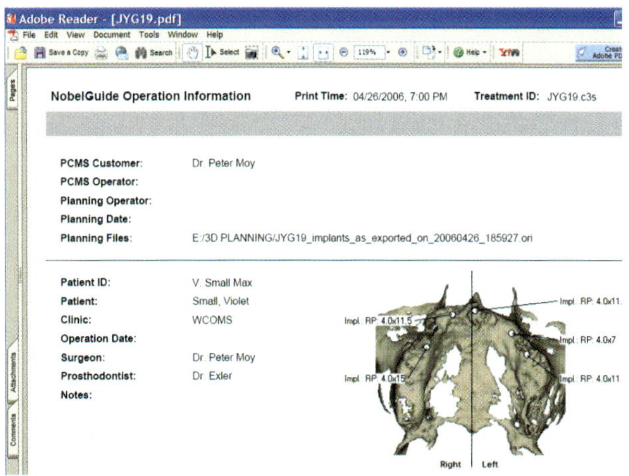

Fig 4-2 (a) Operation information sheet indicating the number and sizes of implants, as well as locations in the alveolar ridge.

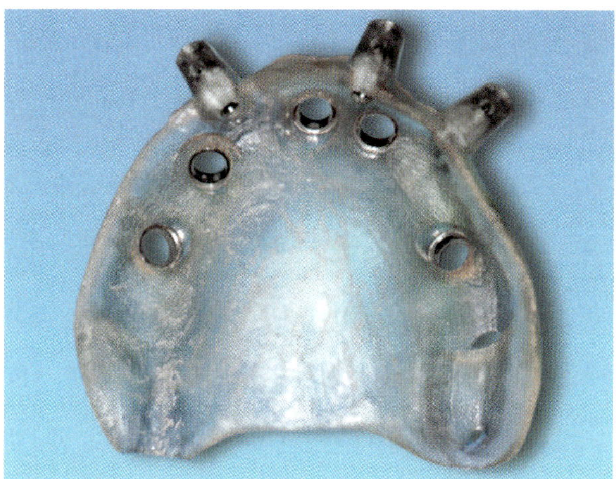

Fig 4-2 (b) Information from the operation information sheet should correspond exactly to the surgical template.

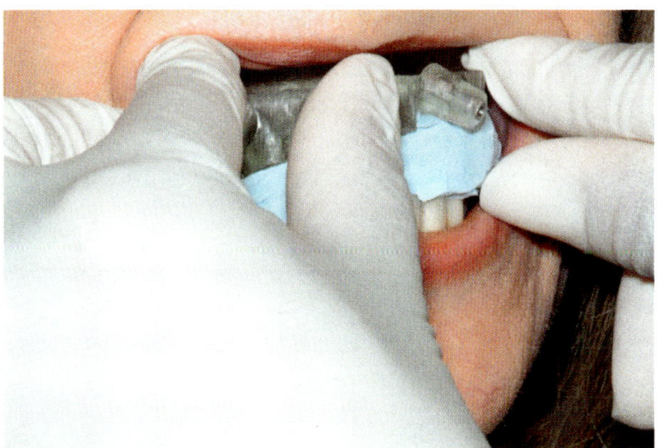

Fig 4-3 (a) The clinician checks the fit of the surgical template to the surgical index, as well as the opposing dentition.

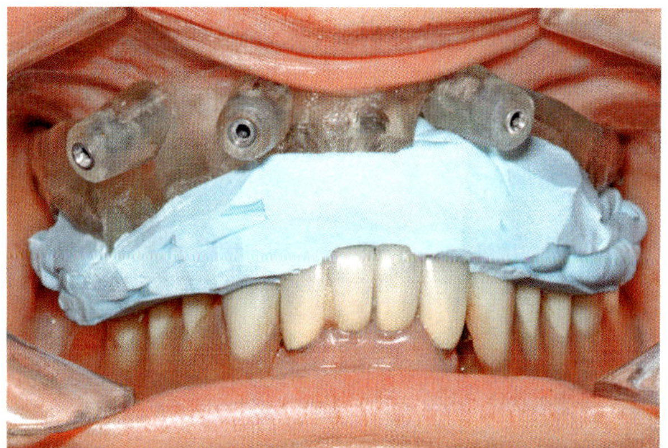

Fig 4-3 (b) Final inspection of the fit prior to initiating drilling procedures. Note the well-fitting surgical index to opposing dentition.

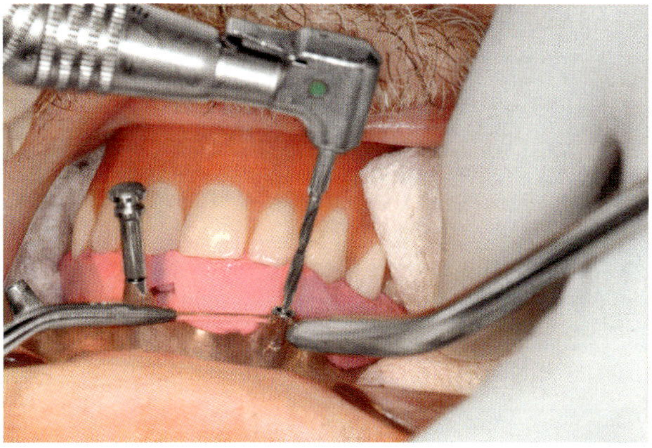

Fig 4-4 (a) Use of a 1.5 mm diameter twist drill through the horizontal guide sleeve. Note that irrigation is applied directly to the entrance of the guide sleeve of the surgical template.

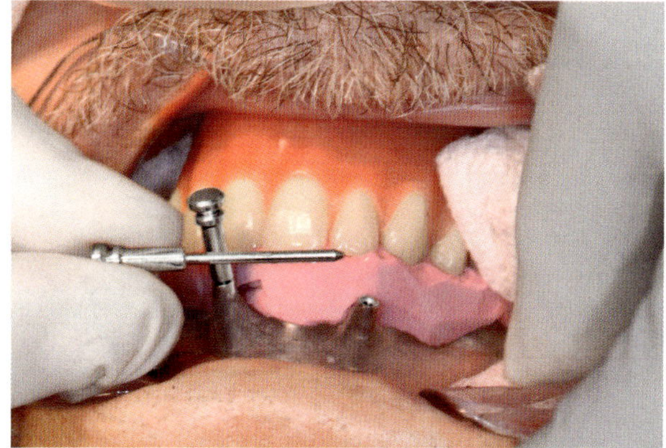

Fig 4-4 (b) Insertion of the horizontal anchor pin for stabilization of the surgical template.

ensuring an optimal fit of the template to the mucosal tissue. The co-operation of the patient is necessary during seating of the surgical template as the patient needs to bite gently into the surgical index to avoid excessive compression of the mucosal tissue by the surgical template. When the

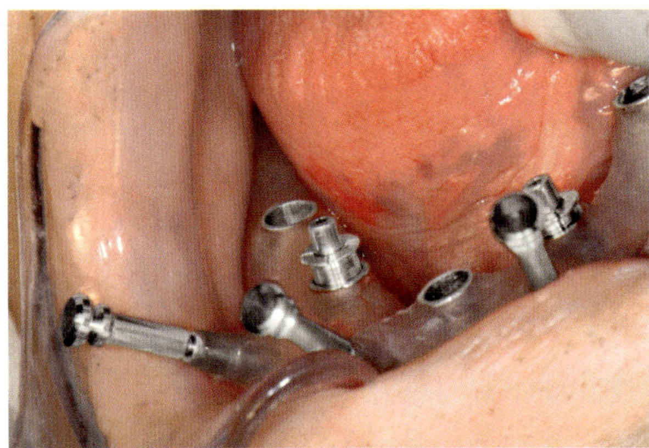

Fig 4-5 The horizontal anchor pins assist in retraction of the lip.

surgical template is fully seated, a 1.5 mm diameter twist drill is used through the horizontal guide sleeve, and a horizontal anchor pin (Fig 4-4a) is inserted to secure the surgical template and prevent it from rotating.

Fully edentulous patients

In the completely edentulous situation, three horizontal anchor pins are used, with one placed around the midline and two posterior, near the commissures of the lip. When the alveolar ridge is severely resorbed and the shape of the ridge is flat, four anchor pins may be necessary to prevent movement of the surgical template (Fig 4-4b). Not only do the anchor pins prevent horizontal movement of the template, but they also assist in retracting the lip (Fig 4-5).

The first two implants placed are known as 'stabilization implants', as these establish the proper vertical compression of the surgical template on the mucosal tissue. The sites for these two implants are the next to the most posterior positions on the surgical template, bilaterally. The drills used to prepare the implant site are designed to remove, slowly and atraumatically, soft tissue and bone, and to avoid heat generation.

The first twist drill is the start drill, which functions as a tissue punch and counterbore. This drill is placed directly into the guide sleeve (Fig 4-6a, b). All subsequent twist drills will have a corresponding drill guide that will fit precisely into the guide sleeve (Fig 4-7a), which prevents the twist drill from wobbling and over-preparing the recipient site. After the start drill, a 2 mm diameter twist drill is used with a 2 mm drill guide (Figs 4-7b, c). Following this, a 3 mm diameter twist drill is used in a corresponding 3 mm drill guide (Fig 4-8a, b). At this point, if the bone is dense, the clinician may use a 3.2 mm diameter twist drill in the 3.2 mm drill guide and finally a screwtap to enlarge the osteotomy site to permit placement of the implant without over-compressing the bone. The tap does not require a guide and is self-centering when the shank contacts the guide sleeve. The recipient bone site is now ready for the implant.

A specially designed implant mount is con-

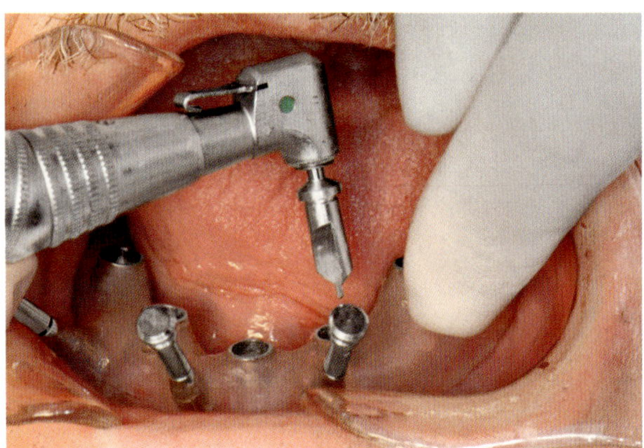

Fig 4-6 (a) The start drill, which combines a tissue punch and countersinking drill, is placed directly into the vertical guide sleeve.

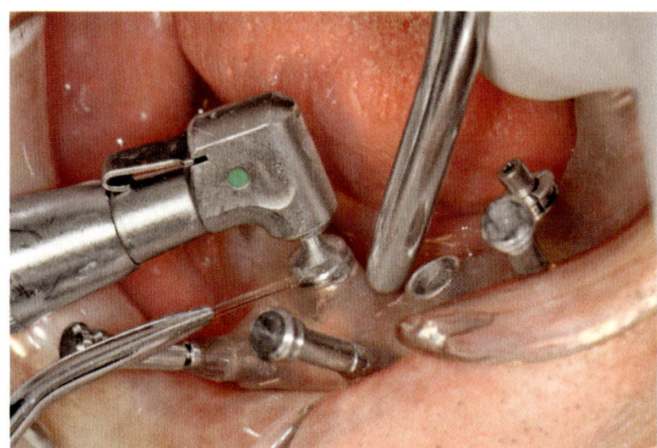

Fig 4-6 (b) Proper use of the start drill requires that the flange on the drill makes full contact with the top of the guide sleeve.

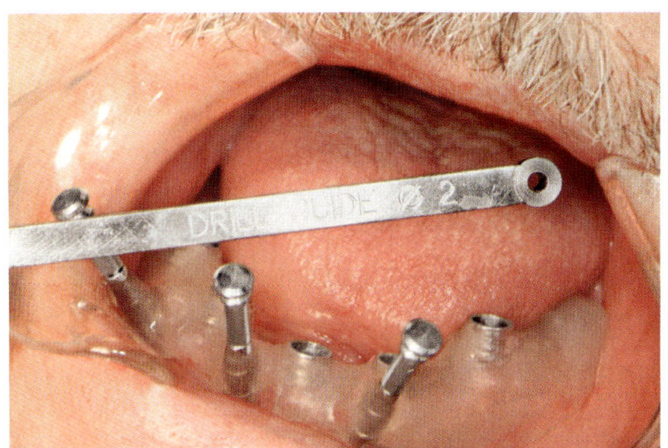

Fig 4-7 (a) A 2 mm drill guide must be used to direct the 2 mm diameter twist drill into the proper position and angulation.

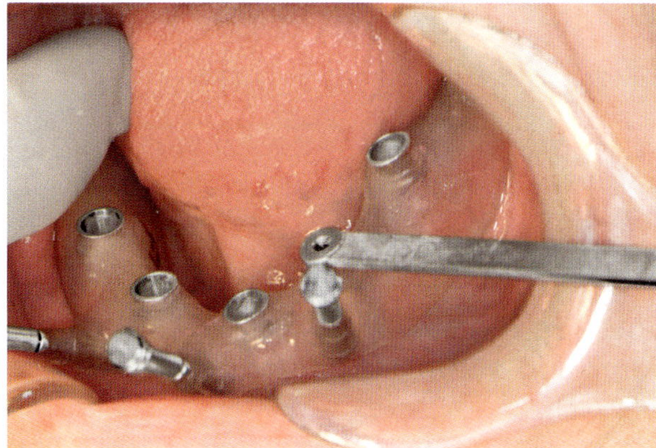

Fig 4-7 (b) The 2 mm drill guide is inserted into the vertical guide sleeve. The clinician must ensure complete seating of the drill guide and contact circumferentially with the guide sleeve.

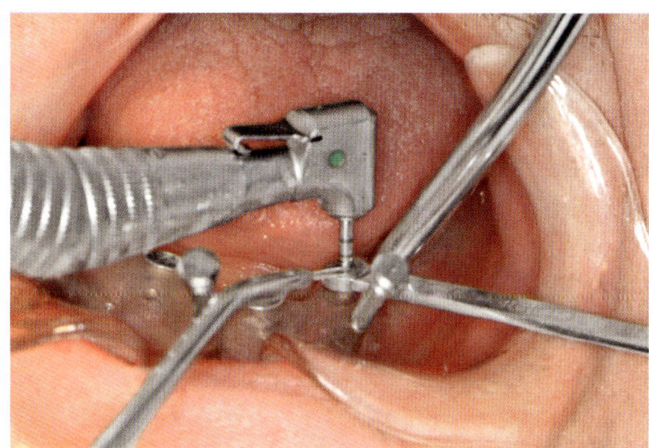

Fig 4-7 (c) The 2 mm twist drill is inserted into the drill guide and is used to prepare the recipient site to the predetermined depth.

nected to the implant and inserted through the guide sleeve to seat the implant (Fig 4-9). The implant mount also self-centers the implant. It is recommended that the two stabilization implants are placed simultaneously and tightened onto the surgical template alternating between the two. This will prevent tipping the surgical template towards the side of the first implant seated, resulting in over-seating of implants on the side that has been compressed. Over-compression of the surgical

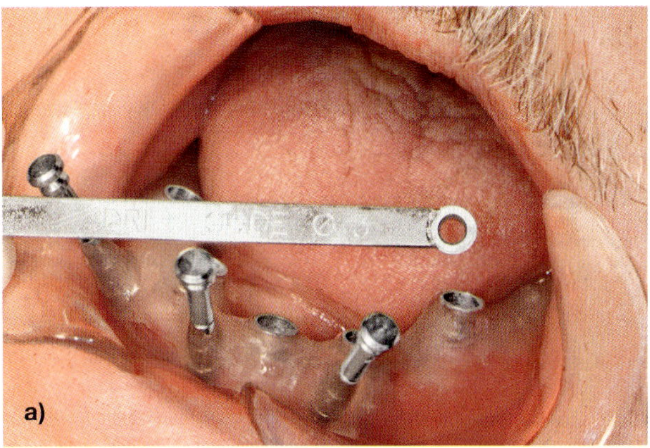

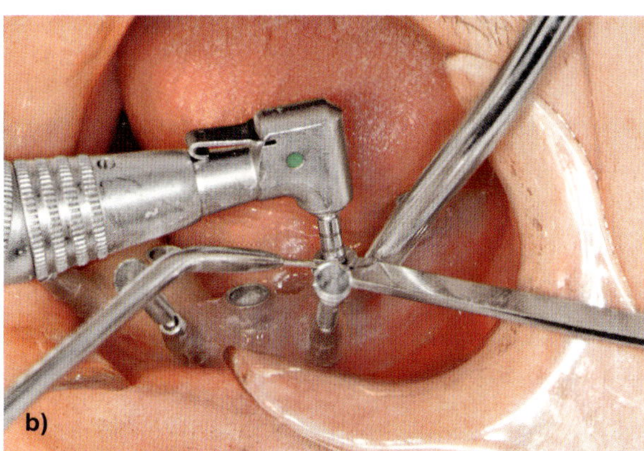

Fig 4-8 (a and b) A 3 mm drill guide is used to direct the 3 mm diameter twist drill.

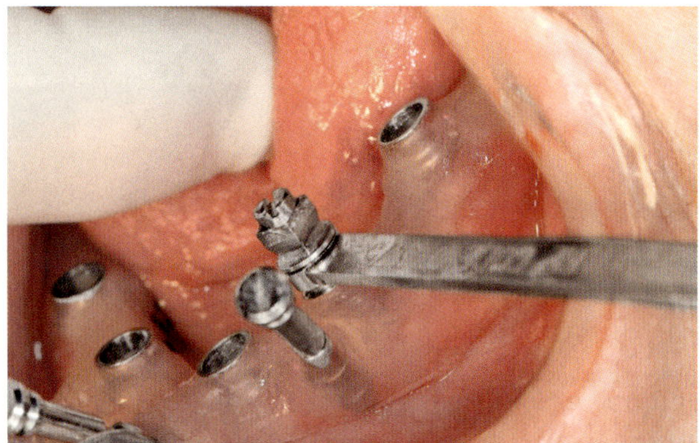

Fig 4-9 To achieve proper vertical seating of the surgical template, the clinician needs to place the two template abutments into the stabilization implants simultaneously. This prevents tipping of the template to one side, maintaining the horizontal plane for placement of the remaining implants.

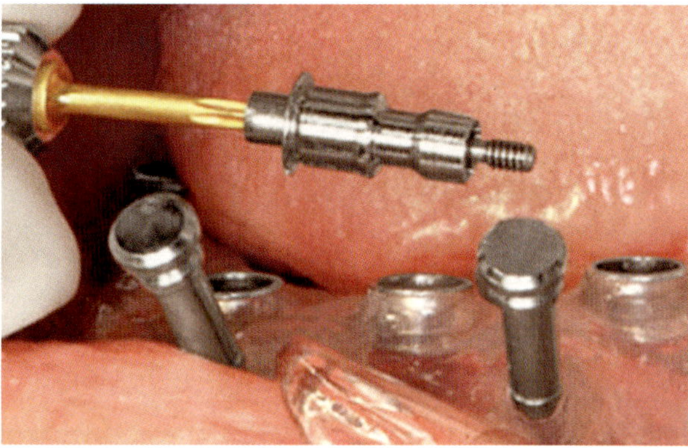

Fig 4-10 (a) The template abutment is specifically designed to avoid over-compression of the surgical template. Slots at the head of the abutment creates four wings, which expand as the abutment screw is tightened into the implant, similar in mechanism to a molly bolt.

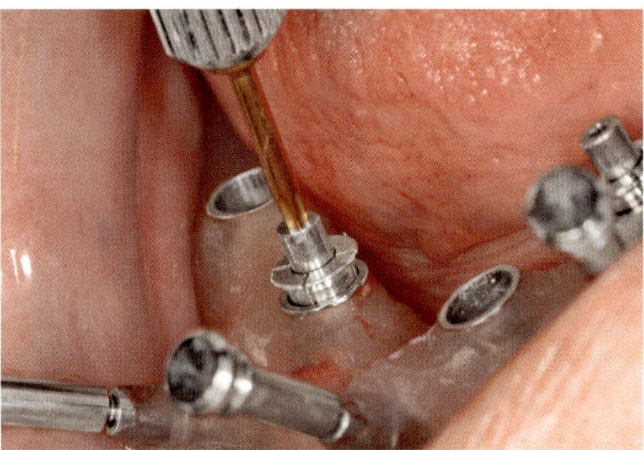

Fig 4-10 (b) Seating of the template abutment is accomplished by slowly tightening the abutment screw into the implant.

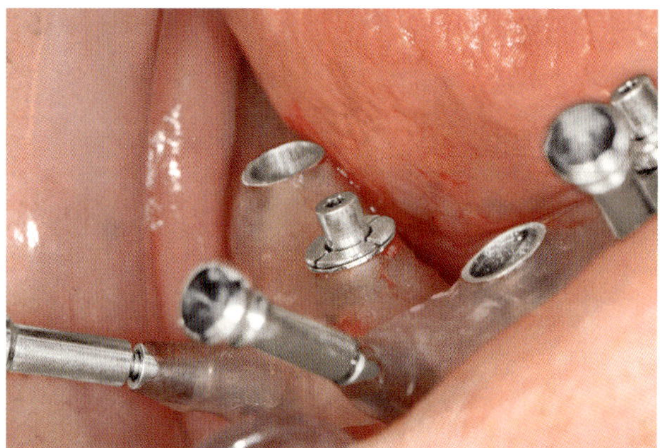

Fig 4-10 (c) During tightening of the abutment screw, the expansion wings of the template abutment applies vertical compression on to the surgical template. The clinician should be certain of complete contact circumferentially between the top of the guide sleeve in the surgical template and the ring of the template abutment.

template on one side may result in a malocclusion with the prefabricated prosthesis. Once stabilization implants are completely seated by confirming that the implant mounts are fully contacting the top of the guide sleeves, the implant mounts are removed and a template abutment (Fig 4-10a to c) is secured to the implants. The template abutment screw head is tapered so that as the screw tightens into the implant it expands the four wings of the abutment in a 'molly bolt' fashion (bolt having tips that expand when the central screw is tightened). The top of the abutment contacts the guide sleeve, and friction is applied laterally as the wings expand against the guide sleeve and as the abutment screw is tightened, thus vertically compressing the surgical template onto the mucosal tissue. The two template abutments should be tightened simultaneously to avoid tipping the surgical template to one side.

After the two stabilization implants are secured with the template abutments, the remaining implant sites are prepared following the sequence of drills described above. Once all implants are placed, the prosthesis is prepared for delivery: the guided abutments are placed into the frame of the prosthesis so that the prosthesis can be inserted as soon as

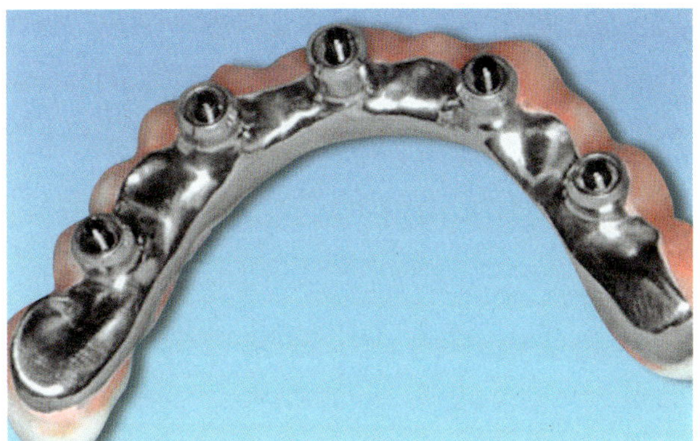

Fig 4-11 Guided abutments have been inserted into the definitive prosthesis, in preparation for connection of the prosthesis to the implants.

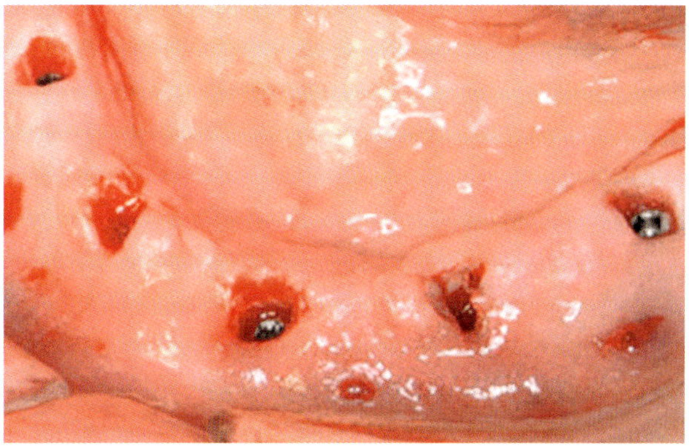

Fig 4-12 The gingival tissue surrounding the head of the implants is removed with a specially designed tissue punch.

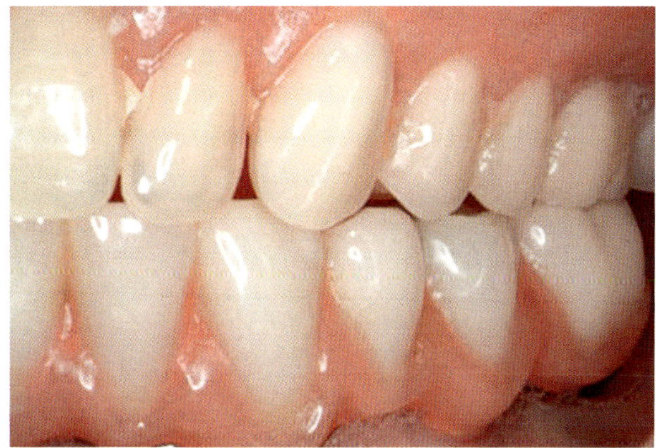

Fig 4-13 The prosthesis should be completely seated onto the implants. Once this is confirmed, the guided abutment screws are tightened with a hand-held torque wrench, and the occlusion in centric and lateral excisions should be carefully checked, as shown.

the surgical template is removed (Fig 4-11). Before the template is removed, a special tissue punch (Fig 4-12) which is designed to fit into the guide sleeves, is used to trim excess gingival tissue. This will allow for easy seating of the prosthesis. The clinician should insert the prosthetic restoration as fast as possible because the surrounding soft tissue has a tendency to collapse, which can create problems for prosthesis insertion.

After all implants have been seated and excess gingival tissue trimmed, the prosthesis can be delivered. Earlier, the surgical–prosthodontic team should have determined which member of the team will place the prosthesis. Clinical experience suggests that the clinician performing surgery is best suited to insert the fixed prosthesis. The clinician has developed a feel for the path of insertion through the placement of the surgical template, placement of implants and fit of surgical components. The delivery of the prosthesis and tightening of the prosthetic screws are performed in a sequential fashion, similar to the placement of implants. Every effort should be made to avoid seating or over-tightening the screws on one side. The guided abutments work similarly to the template abutments. There are four wings at the top of the guided abutment that expand as the abutment screw is tightened into the implant. Once the wings of the abutment screw expand, there is friction against the prosthetic frame preventing the prosthesis from sliding vertically along the length of the abutment. Therefore, the abutment screws should be tightened to where the tip of the screw is just engaging the internal threads of the implant. Once all abutment screws are engaging the implants, the patient is asked to close down gently into the prosthesis. A few tapping, closure movements by the patient will assist in seating the prosthesis evenly and locating the proper vertical dimension of occlusion for the patient.

When all abutment screws have been hand-tightened, a radiograph should be taken to confirm that all guided abutments are seated completely on to the tops of the implants. After confirmation that the prosthesis is completely seated into the implants, the abutment screws are tightened to 35 Ncm using the hand-held torque wrench.

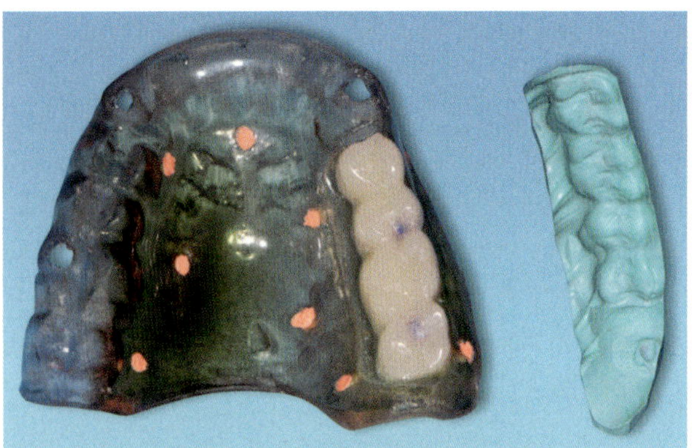

Fig 4-14 Palatal view of a radiographic guide, showing the positions of radiopaque markers placed into the palatal vault. The placement of these markers helps to avoid the potential overlapping of images of the markers with endodontically treated root apices in partially dentate patients.

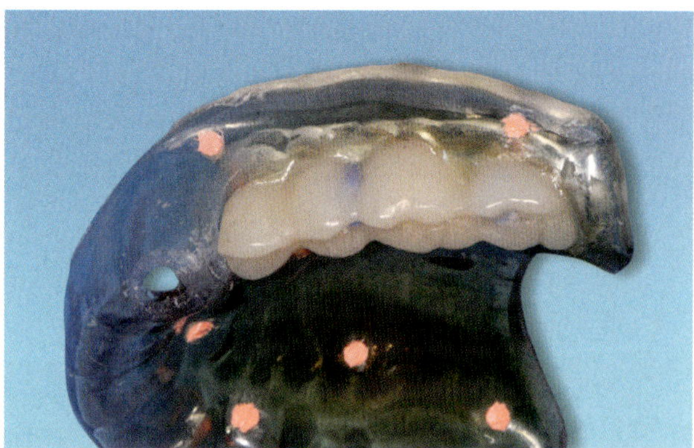

Fig 4-15 A radiographic guide designed specifically for the partially dentate patient. Note the 'observation window' created in the cusp tip of the canine.

Once the prosthesis is inserted, the prosthodontist should carefully check the occlusion in centric and lateral excursions to avoid any excessive load on implants (Fig 4-13). Special care should also be taken to manage the embrasures to allow adequate hygiene and maintenance. Esthetics, speech and comfort are achievable using NobelGuide flapless surgery.

Partially dentate patients

In partially dentate and single-missing tooth situations, the clinician must make a decision as to the cost-effectiveness and usefulness of using software planning (Procera) versus a model-based planning workup. A contraindication to using computer-based planning may be found if the adjacent dentition in the partially dentate state has metal restorations or endodontic treatment; this is because radiopaque materials could create scatter or block the radiopaque markers in the radiographic guide. Scatter caused by metal restorations will reduce the accuracy of computerized tomography and often block the view of the bony anatomy. Endodontic filler material will block visualization of the radiopaque markers placed into the radiographic guide. When this occurs, the planning software program will not be able to convert the DICOM files, thus rendering the scans useless. A minimum of four radiopaque markers must be visualized before the planning program can superimpose the markers from the two scans. This limitation is found with the older version of the software. The newest version of Procera software (version 2.0) will permit conversion of the DICOM files without the presence of the radiopaque markers.

The partially dentate patient workup, radiographic guide, and surgical template have slight differences from the completely edentulous patient. The workup must take into consideration adjacent root structures and metal restorations. These findings will dictate where the radiopaque markers are placed on the radiographic guide and whether horizontal anchor pin(s) are used. If there is a possibility that intraoral structures will mask the markers, it is recommended that the markers should be placed high into the palatal vault or deep into the lingual and/or buccal vestibule, beyond the apices of the roots (Fig 4-14). The radiographic guide is shaped differently for the partially dentate patient. The guide should just cover the incisal and occlusal surfaces of natural dentition present and replicate, but not cover, occlusal surfaces of the pontics exactly.

In the partially dentate patient, the radiographic guide and surgical template contains inspection windows cut through the incisal or occlusal surfaces (Fig 4-15). These openings in the template

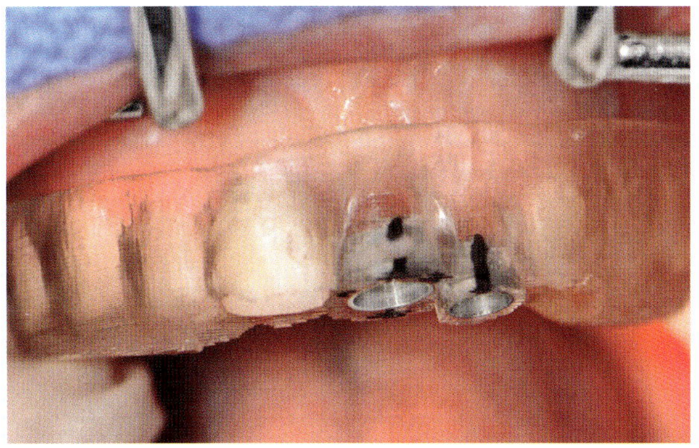

Fig 4-16 The windows will allow, during the surgery, control of the perfect setting of the surgical guide.

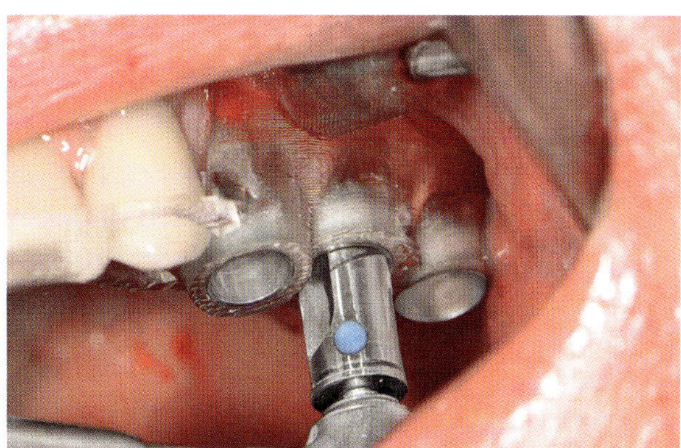

Fig 4-17 The implants being placed: the guide should remain stable, in order for the optimal fit to be controlled through the windows.

permit the clinician to visualize and ensure that the template is seated completely on to the teeth (Figs 16 and 17). With limited mesial-to-distal spacing, if adjacent root structures are close to the edentulous space, or when using model-based planning, the horizontal anchor pin is not used. This is to avoid damaging roots or reducing the available bone to support the implants. Stabilization of the surgical template is achieved by engaging the natural dentition and with the stabilization implant(s). Other than these variations from the protocol, the surgical steps are essentially the same for the partially dentate states as for the completely edentulous.

The clinician may want to change one aspect of guided surgery when operating in the esthetic zone of partially dentate patients. When gingival biotype is thin, the tissue punch or a flapless approach should be avoided. A minimal-flap procedure is used to avoid undesired removal of tissue; this approach also controls excessive contraction and recession of the marginal tissue around the immediate loaded implant, and the adjacent natural dentition. A minimal-flap procedure allows for better control of the repositioned flap to place the attached tissue where it is needed; in some clinical situations, a minimal-flap procedure enables re-establishment of interproximal papilla (see Chapter 5 for a discussion of the papillae regeneration technique). When gingival contours are deficient or of poor gingival biotype, the use of guided surgery in the esthetic zone is contraindicated. The clinician must be ready to perform open-flap surgery and take other prosthodontic measures to provide the patient with immediate loading in the esthetic zone.

Postoperative patient instructions

The patient should be instructed to remain on a soft, 'non-chewing' diet for a minimum of 2 weeks. By focusing on a non-chewing diet, the patient will be acutely aware of the need to avoid chewing with the newly placed implant and restoration. Other routine post-surgical instructions that should be given are use of ice to minimize swelling, warm saline rinses and oral hygiene instructions. The follow-up schedule is extremely important. At each post-surgical visit, inspection of occlusion with articulating paper should be performed. Occlusion changes dramatically once the local anesthetic has worn off and the patient starts to feel comfortable with the fixed restorative prosthesis, as there is typically very little pain or discomfort. During this critical period, heavy occlusal contacts must be reduced and, most importantly, lateral interferences eliminated. Lateral prematurities are the most detrimental force on immediate load implants and lead to early failure of the implant.

Part II: NobelGuide, zygoma implants and immediate function

Introduction to zygoma implants

Oral rehabilitation with implants is well documented and many protocols have been developed to simplify procedures for the clinician, the prosthodontist and the patient. Many solutions have been provided to enhance the esthetic and functional aspects of reconstruction of the maxilla.

Oxidized surface of implants promotes faster bone formation (Glauser et al 2002, Ivanoff et al 2003), increasing primary stability and responds more effectively to demanding situations, such as soft or deficient bone in the maxilla. Severe resorption of the posterior maxilla can jeopardize rehabilitation of fully edentulous patients by means of implants.

Good results have been published with short implants placed in the posterior maxilla (Renouard and Nisand 2005).

Nevertheless, rehabilitation of the posterior maxilla where bone volume is insufficient, i.e. less than 5 mm, remains a challenge. Poor anchorage owing to insufficient height or width of bone has previously led to the need for additional therapies, such as apposition bone grafting, sinus graft and osteogenesis distraction (Jensen 2006).

Sinus grafting is a well-known and popular procedure. Despite this, bone augmentation and the insertion of implants with or without immediate loading offers success rates between 60 and 98% (Wallace and Froum 2003). Using implants with oxidized surfaces considerably improves the success rates of these procedures (Lundgren and Brechter 2002). However some patients may be reluctant to undergo such procedures.

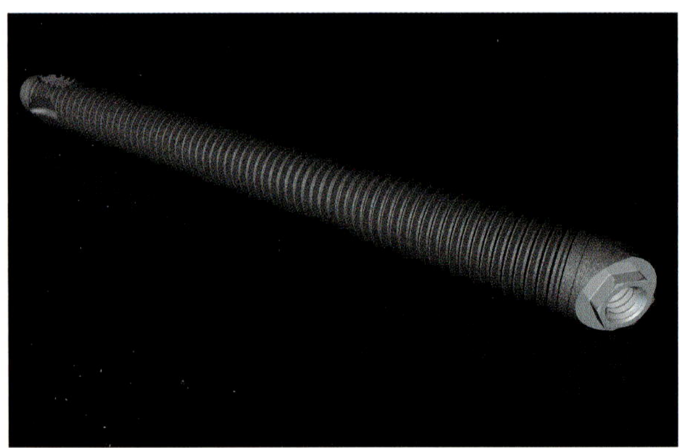

Fig 4-18 zygoma implant with a TiUnite surface.

To avoid bone grafting, other solutions have been proposed: tilted implants placed in the tuberosity or the pterygoid plate, and implants following the anterior sinus wall, diminishing the cantilever applied to the fixed prosthesis (Aparicio et al 2001, 2002, Calandriello and Tomatis 2005).

Inserting implants in the pterygoid process is demanding because this technique has been associated with the risk of causing injury to the descending maxillary vasculature (Choi and Park 2003).

To address the problem of very poor bone volume, zygoma implants have proven to be successful in supporting fixed prostheses without bone grafting (Bedrossian et al 2002, Malevez et al 2004). The use of zygoma implants compensates for insufficiencies in poor maxillary structures by an anchorage in the zygoma.

Zygoma implants are available in different lengths: 30, 35, 40, 42.5, 45, 47.5, 50 and 52.5 mm. There are two diameters, 3.9 mm at the top and 4.6 mm at the level of the maxilla where it has an angulation of 45° corresponding to the angulation of the zygoma with the maxilla (Fig 4-18). These implants are used even if the maxillary height is less than 5 mm.

Any edentulous maxillary situation can be treated using zygoma implants. The zygomatic anchorage is very strong and these long implants have a high success rate. Zygoma implants can be placed in addition to two, three or four anterior standard implants (Fig 4-19).

If the anterior remaining maxillary bone is less than 7 mm, four zygoma implants can also be sufficient for supporting a totally fixed prosthesis (Fig 4-20).

Zygoma implants can also benefit immediate loading (Bedrossian et al 2006). As with standard implants, their oxidized surface enhances osseointegration.

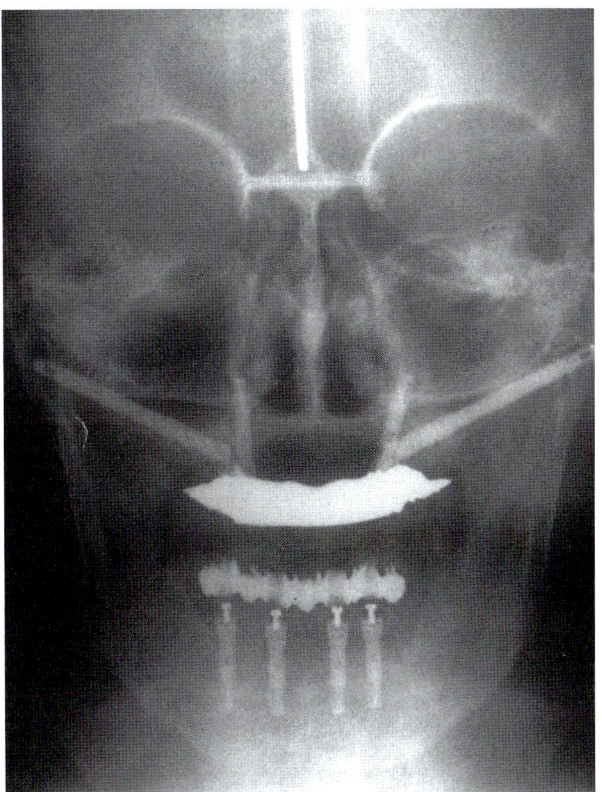

Fig 4-19 Facial image of two zygoma implants and two standard implants in the canine region with a fixed Procera Implant Bridge.

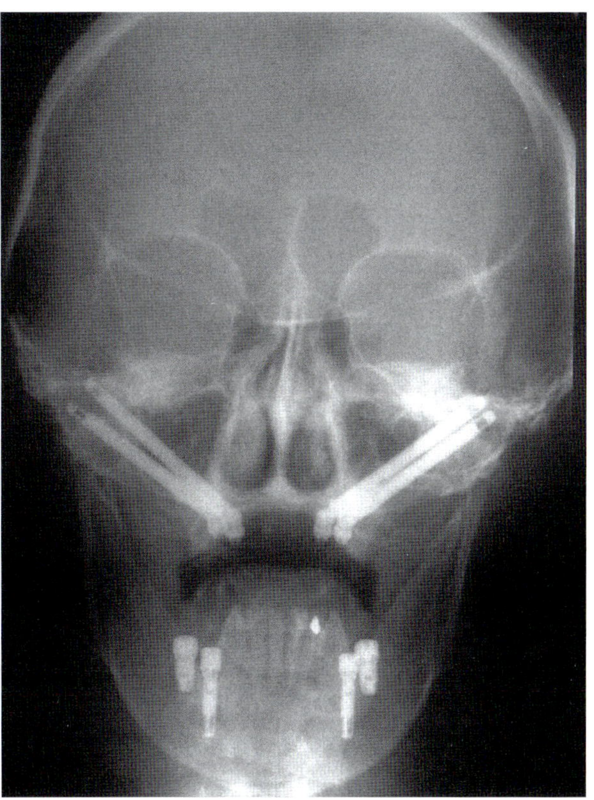

Fig 4-20 Placement of four zygoma implants for supporting a fixed prosthesis.

Surgical standard protocol

The standard protocol for inserting zygoma implants involves opening a wide mucoperiosteal flap to uncover the maxilla as well as the anterior sinus wall up to the zygomatic incisura. This enables viewing of the total sinus wall and zygoma (Fig 4-21).

Although the associated pain is moderate, the patient can experience swelling and discomfort for days following the surgery. Despite that, a provisional prosthesis can be installed immediately; this therapy requires an impression to be taken at the time of surgery and careful adjustment of the occlusion. The creation of a definitive prosthesis is also required some months later. The ideal placement of implants and the need for minimally invasive surgery are challenges, but zygoma implants provide an appropriate solution for performing implant therapy.

Zygoma implants and NobelGuide

The NobelGuide concept allows insertion of implants with guided surgery by means of presurgical computerized preparation. The Teeth-in-an-Hour procedure involves insertion of the definitive prosthesis at the time of the surgery. This procedure is currently being developed for zygoma implants using a special surgical guide and hardware for inserting the implants in the right position. This enables immediate placement of the definitive prosthesis.

After computerized tomography up to the level of the zygoma together with the radiological guide, Procera software enables virtual positioning of the zygoma implants and the realization of a fixed prosthesis (Procera Implant Bridge). A special surgical guide is made for drilling and insertion of the zygoma implants. Special hardware with sleeves of different diameters is available. It is

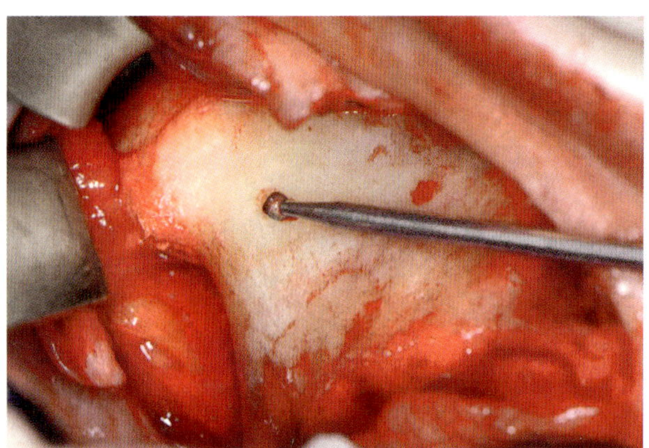

Fig 4-21 The whole mucosa is reflected, showing the maxilla up to the top of the zygoma. The drill indicates the sinus window.

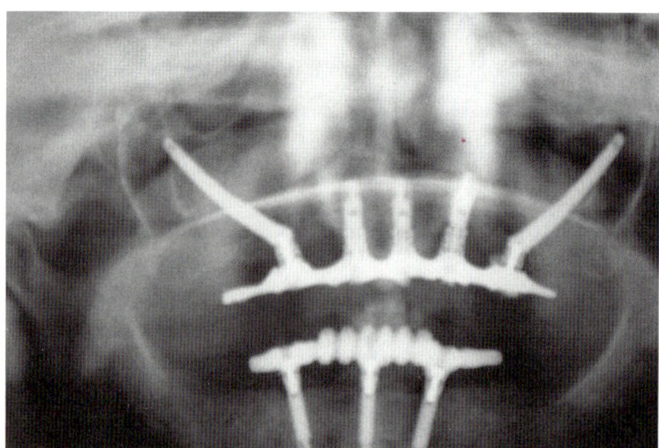

Fig 4-22 Orthopantomogram 1 month post-surgery.

essential that zygoma implants are placed with a guide because of their length and the need for precise positioning.

After insertion in the mouth, the surgical guide is fixed with three to four pins. Drilling starts with the standard implants following the NobelGuide protocol. Next, a 2.9 mm calibrated drill inserted in a special sleeve is used to prepare the site of the zygoma implants, and then a second drill of 3.6 mm diameter and a counterbore are used.

At the maxillary level of the zygoma implant, two openings are made through the mucosa: one for the implant and one for viewing the screw of the original fixture mount, which will indicate the exact position of the angulated head.

The zygoma implant is then fixed on a second fixture mount, which is screwed on the first one; this helps to indicate the moment when insertion should be stopped. The wide fixture mount will be inserted in a sleeve to guide the implant up to the top of the zygoma.

After insertion of all the implants, the surgical guide is removed and the prosthesis is inserted. It is screwed on the anterior implants and cemented on the posterior ones.

Advantages of this procedure are that there is no incision, no stitches, no swelling and treatment time is shortened. Insertion of the implants as well as the prosthesis can be performed in 1 hour 15 minutes and immediate function is realized by means of a definitive prosthesis.

No chairside impression or bite registration is required after the surgery, as the prosthesis is prepared beforehand and inserted during surgery.

Conclusion

The development of zygoma implants used in conjunction with the NobelGuide concept highlights the possibility of rehabilitating patients with total edentulism and insufficient bone volume by means of minimally invasive surgery and immediate reconstruction of their masticatory function (Figs 4-22 and 4-23).

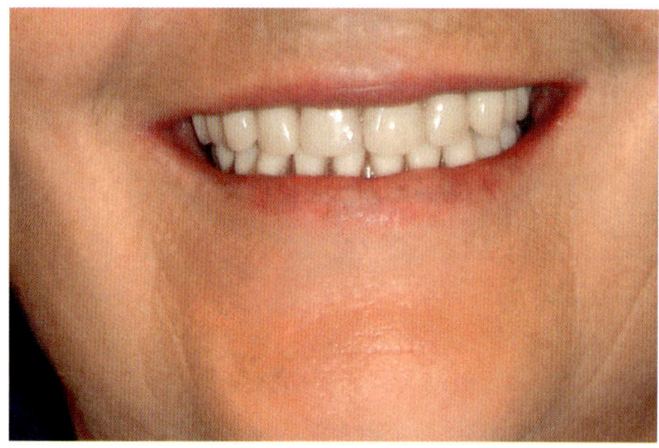

Fig 4-23 The prosthesis placed on the day of surgery.

References

Aparicio C, Arévalo JX, Ouazzani W, Granados C. Retrospective clinical and radiographic evaluation of tilted implants used in the treatment of the severely resorbed edentulous maxilla. Appl Osseointegration Res 2002;3:17-21

Aparicio C, Perales P, Rangert B. Tilted implants as an alternative to maxillary sinus grafting: a clinical, radiologic, and Periotest study. Clin Implants Dent Relat Res 2001;3:39-49.

Bedrossian E, Stumpel LJ. The zygomatic implant: preliminary data on treatment of severely resorbed maxillae. A clinical report. Int J Oral Maxillofac Implants 2002;17:861-865.

Bedrossian E, Rangert B, Stumpel L, Indersano T. Immediate function with the zygomatic implant. A graftless solution for the patient with mild to advanced atrophy of the maxilla. Int J Oral Maxillofac Implants 2006;21:937-942.

Calandriello R, Tomatis M. Simplified treatment of the atrophic posterior maxilla via immediate/early function and tilted implants: a prospective 1-year clinical study. Clin Implants Dent Relat Res 2005;7(Suppl 1):S1-S12.

Choi J, Park HS. The clinical anatomy of the maxillary artery in the pterygopalatine fossa. J Oral Maxillofac Surg 2003;61:72-78.

Ericsson I, Nilson H, Nilner K. Immediate functional loading of Brånemark single tooth implants. A 5-year clinical follow-up study. Appl Osseointegration Res 2001;2:12-16.

Glauser R, Portmann M, Ruhstaller P, Lundgren AK, Hammerle CHF, Gottlow J. Stability measurements of immediately loaded machined and oxidized implants in the posterior maxilla. A comparative clinical study using resonance frequency analysis. Appl Osseointegration Res 2001;2:27-29.

Glauser R, Schupbach P, Lundgen AK, Gottlow J, Hämmerle CHF. Machined and oxidized micro-implants retrieved from humans: a comparison using histomorphometry and micro-computed tomography. Clin Oral Implants Res 2002;13:4.

Horiuchi K, Uchida H, Yamamoto K, Sugimura M. Immediate loading of Brånemark system implants following alcement in edentulous atients: A clinical report. Int J Oral Maxillofac Implants 2000;15:824-830.

Ivanoff CJ, Widmark G, Johansson C, Wennerberg A. Histologic evaluation of bone response to oxidized and turned titanium micro-implants in human jawbone. Int J Oral Maxillofac Implants 2003;18:341-348.

Jensen OT. The sinus bone graft, 2nd edition. Chicago: Quintessence, 2006.

Lundgren S, Brechter M. Preliminary findings of using oxidized titanium implants in reconstructive jaw surgery. Appl Osseointegration Res 2002;3:35-39.

Malevez C, Abarca M, Durdu F, Daelemans P. Clinical outcome of 103 consecutive zygomatic implants: a 6-48 months follow-up study. Clin Oral Implants Res 2004;15:18-22.

Renouard F, Nisand D. Short implants in the severely resorbed maxilla: a 2-year retrospective clinical study. Clin Implant Dent Relat Res 2005;(Suppl 1):S104-S110.

Wallace SS, Froum SJ. Effect of maxillary sinus augmentation on the survival of endosseous dental implants. A systematic review. Ann Periodontol 2003;8:328-343.

Chapter 5

Esthetic considerations

Patrick Palacci

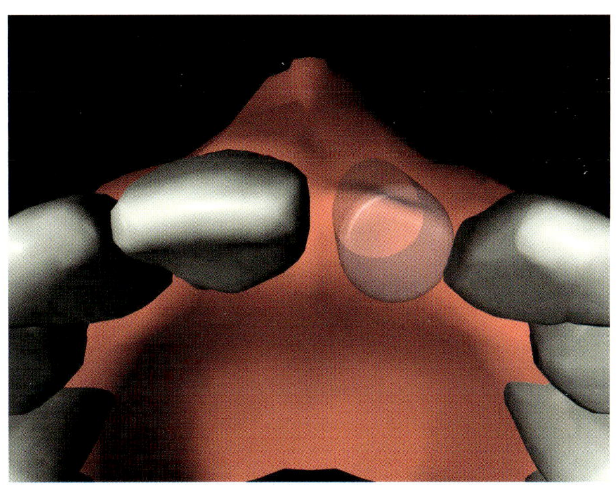

General principles

According to the needs and the wishes of the patients, implant treatment should include esthetics as an important consideration. Although the patient will receive a temporary or final prosthesis just after the surgery, this does not diminish the importance of esthetics. The clinician and prosthodontist need to be aware that this procedure is usually definitive. When dealing with two-stage surgery, one-stage surgery and delayed loading, the clinician can manage hard and soft tissue at each different stage to achieve the final optimal result.

Implant placement and angulation strongly influence the final functional, biomechanical and esthetic results, especially in the partially edentulous patient. The NobelGuide concept allows the clinician to achieve this goal by optimizing implant placement. However, when using this concept and dealing with flapless surgery, every surgical step is oriented towards optimal implant positioning according to the prosthetic restoration, assuming that this positioning is achievable with no additive surgery and that the soft tissue contour will not undergo further change. The clinician should carefully evaluate the patient from an esthetic point of view and evaluate hard and soft tissue quality and quantity. The patient's preferences should also be taken into account.

Fully edentulous patients

In most cases, treatment of fully edentulous patients does not require hard and soft tissue manipulation to optimize the final esthetic result. Bone loss is generally such that successful esthetics can be achieved with lip support and by using the smile line as a guide, rather than soft tissue anatomy. Lip support and the 'pink esthetic' will be obtained by the porcelain or acrylic gingival replacement included in the prosthesis. This material will compensate for bone loss and lack of superior lip support. In addition, flapless surgery minimizes trauma and there is very little or even no soft tissue modification.

During pre-prosthetic and pre-surgical evaluations, the clinician can have an exact idea of the final anatomy and then decide on the almost definitive shape of the prosthesis according to the selected implant positioning. The prosthetic contour should be designed to avoid lack of lip support, lack of black triangles, speech problems and food impaction.

These factors can be analyzed on the model before implant surgery and addressed before implant positioning (Figs 5-1 and 5-2). The practitioner can adapt the prosthesis to the future clinical situation by knowing exactly where implants will be placed. However, there may be some significant differences between the facial esthetics

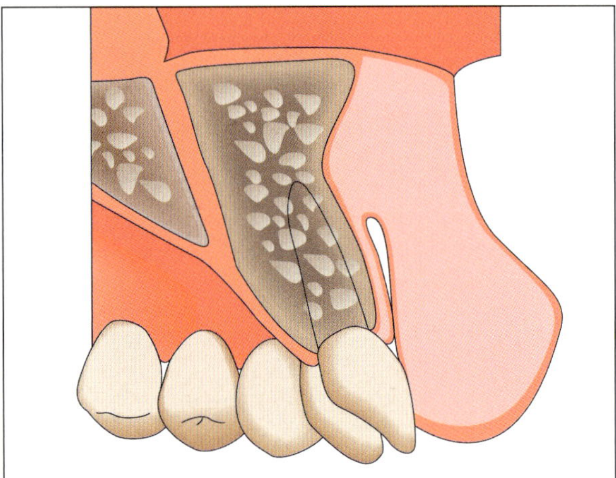

Fig 5-1 Healthy clinical situation with the anterior teeth in place as well as a normal bone ridge. Note the optimal lip support.

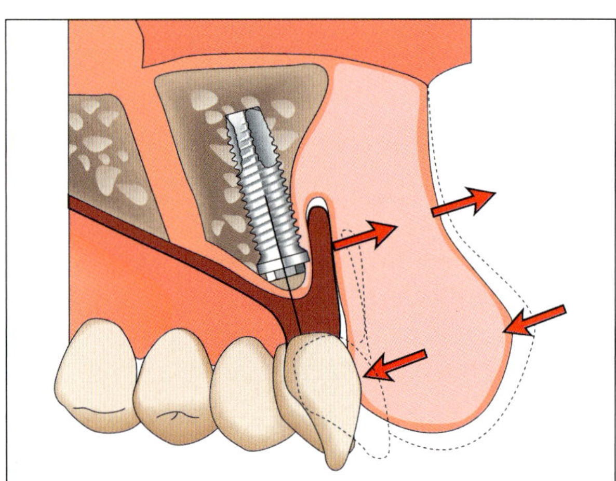

Fig 5-2 In an edentulous situation with significant ridge resorption, a denture is fabricated. The labial flange of the prosthesis is responsible for a subsnasal convexity and loss of labial edge.

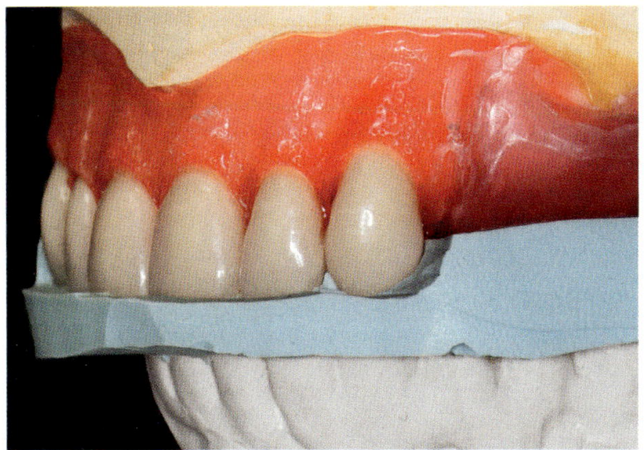

Fig 5-3 To determine precisely the end result, the labial flange should be removed in the anterior region from cuspid to cuspid when trying in the teeth. The teeth will be probably placed in a more labial position to gain lip support and to compensate for the lack of labial flange.

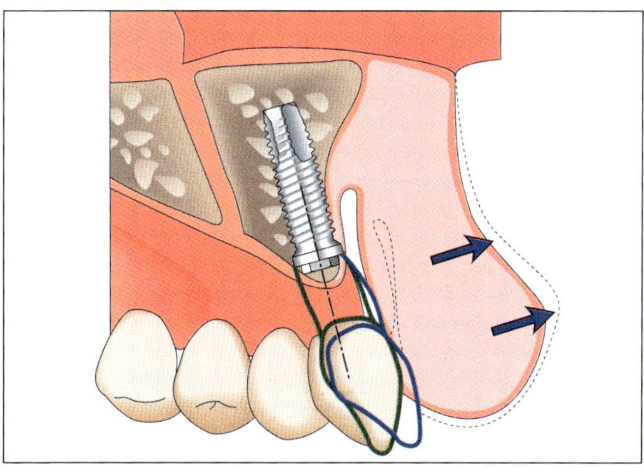

Fig 5-4 Final prosthesis is in place, illustrating that a labial flange is not necessary to obtain adequate lip support. Position of the teeth is critical for esthetic success.

obtained with the esthetic model base and the final result with the fixed prosthesis in place (Figs 5-3 and 5-4)

The esthetic model base must have a high labial flange to obtain a perfect fit and to position the stabilization pins on the surgical guide. This flange will push the tissues labially just below the nose, and the lip will consequently collapse. If the final position of the teeth is similar to the esthetic model base, there will be a significant lack of support of the lip. To avoid this complication, the esthetic model base should be first fabricated without the labial flange and the esthetic should then be determined at this stage of the procedure.

Once the correct positioning has been confirmed, the flange is added to the model base and the clinician follows the normal protocol. When placing the fixed partial denture, especially on the maxilla, some adaptation problems may occur. As the patient is likely to have been wearing a denture previously, the patient can sometimes experience discomfort, airflow and speech problems with this new prosthesis in place.

To avoid these complications, the prosthesis should be fabricated with an excess of acrylic nearly filling all the spaces between the implants for at least a week (Fig 5-5).

The patient will then accommodate to this new situation with a fixed prosthesis and no palate.

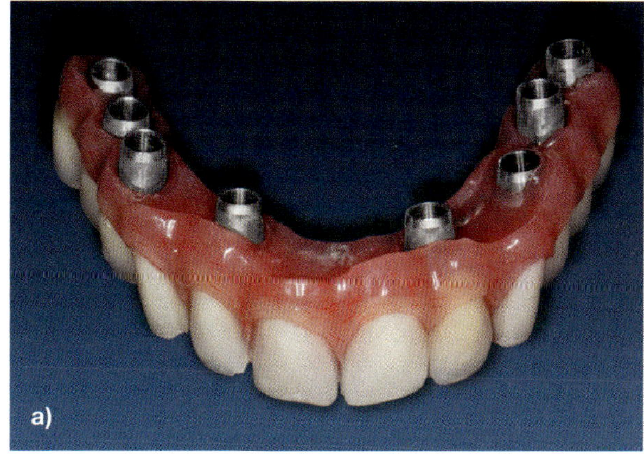

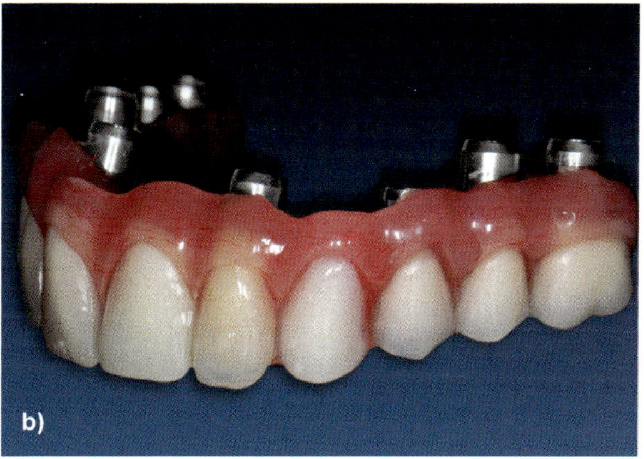

Fig 5-5 (a and b) The temporary restoration is fabricated with an excess of acrylic material at the ridge level.

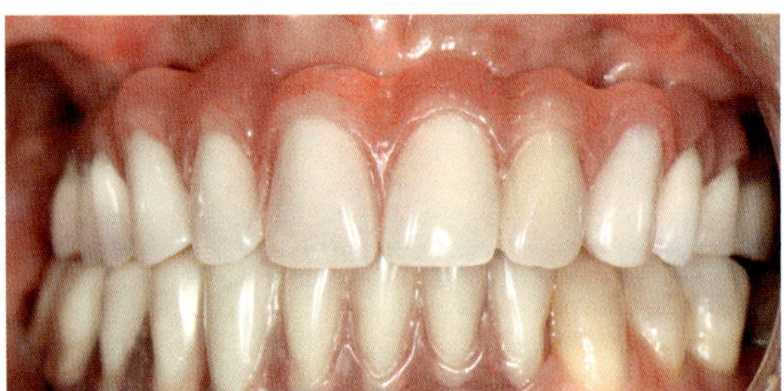

Fig 5-6 After a week, the pink acrylic is reshaped to promote hygiene and to avoid speech problems. After 3 months, the prosthetic restoration is re-evaluated and the embrasures are modified according to the ridge remodeling.

Then the embrasures should be created to allow the optimal combination between maintenance and hygiene, and speech and esthetics.

To avoid complications, according to the esthetics and expectations of the patients, it may be preferable in certain cases to begin with a temporary fixed restoration, to check all the parameters (esthetics, vertical dimension, occlusion, phonetics, hygiene and emergence profile) and then, several months later, to fabricate a definitive Procera Implant Bridge taking into account all of these factors (Figs 5-6 to 5-8).

Partially edentulous patients

Problems related to partially edentulous patients are significantly more complex than for the fully edentulous patient. As implant positioning and soft tissue contour will be definitive using NobelGuide, special care is needed when treating these patients.

All information should be obtained before the treatment starts. This will include information about ridge shape and bone quantity and quality, as well as:

- number, shape and position of the adjacent and opposing teeth
- occlusion
- soft tissue quality and quantity
- color, texture and shape of tissues
- presence or absence of papillæ
- smile line and lip mobility
- personal needs of the patient and psychological factors.

All these factors need to be evaluated, as this surgery can be considered definitive if using the flapless (tissue-punch) technique.

With two-stage surgery, hard and/or soft tissue anatomy can be modified using different additive procedures, but these cannot be modified when choosing the NobelGuide option using the flapless basic protocol.

All these factors have to be evaluated, and pre-implant surgery may be required to achieve the optimal esthetic result.

Before commencing treatment, the clinician should evaluate which is the optimal treatment. In some instances, the ridge seems adequate and a tissue-punch technique may be appropriate for

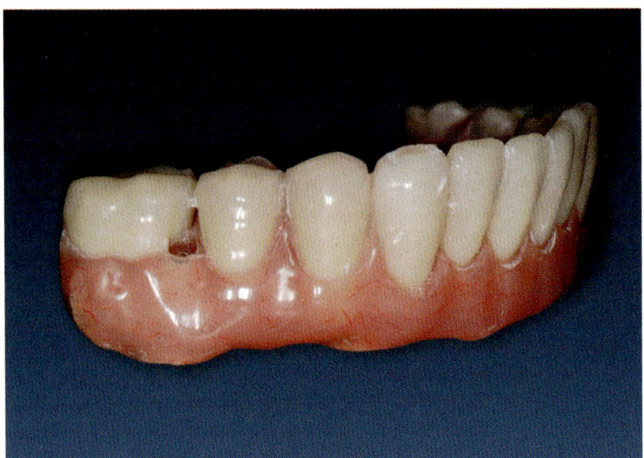

Fig 5-7 The same protocol (as seen in Figs 5-5 and 5-6) is followed in the lower arch. The final prosthesis is now ready to be placed.

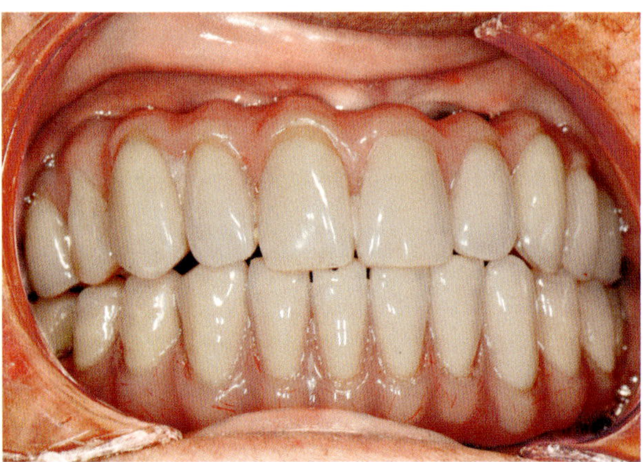

Fig 5-8 Clinical view of a Procera Implant Bridge in the upper and lower arch after 1 year.

esthetics, or there may be a lack of tissue but the esthetic needs are not very high (e.g. when there is a low lip line and low lip mobility). In both of these cases, the conventional protocol may have a satisfactory result.

In other situations, there can be significant ridge resorption (hard and/or soft tissue). In such cases, the clinician has to decide which treatment to choose from the following options.

- A preliminary hard/soft tissue augmentation and treatment using NobelGuide after a healing period.
- Application of the NobelGuide concept with a modified surgical technique using a flap surgical technique together with a papillæ regeneration technique.
- Avoid treating the patient using this technique if, for example, there is limited space between teeth or between teeth and implants. The sleeve of the guide can be a limiting factor if there is a limited space in height and a limited space between implants; there may be difficulty with inserting the guide, and optimal implant placement may be compromised. For these reasons the following four aspects should be carefully evaluated:
  - hard tissue
  - soft tissue
  - prosthetic restorations
  - esthetic requirements.

To select adequate surgical options, the classification described by Palacci and Ericsson in 2001 is of great help to the clinician, prosthodontist and general practitioner in determining the commencement and completion time of the defined treatment. Following is a brief summary of the classification to clarify the treatment approach in relation to esthetics.

Esthetic anterior maxilla classification

This anterior maxilla classification is based on the amount of vertical and horizontal loss of hard and soft tissues. It is divided into four classes according to vertical and horizontal dimensions of these two types of tissue.

Vertical loss (Fig 5-9)

Class I: intact or slightly reduced papillæ
Class II: limited loss of papillæ (less than 50% of papillæ loss)
Class III: severe loss of papillæ
Class IV: absence of papillæ (edentulous ridge).

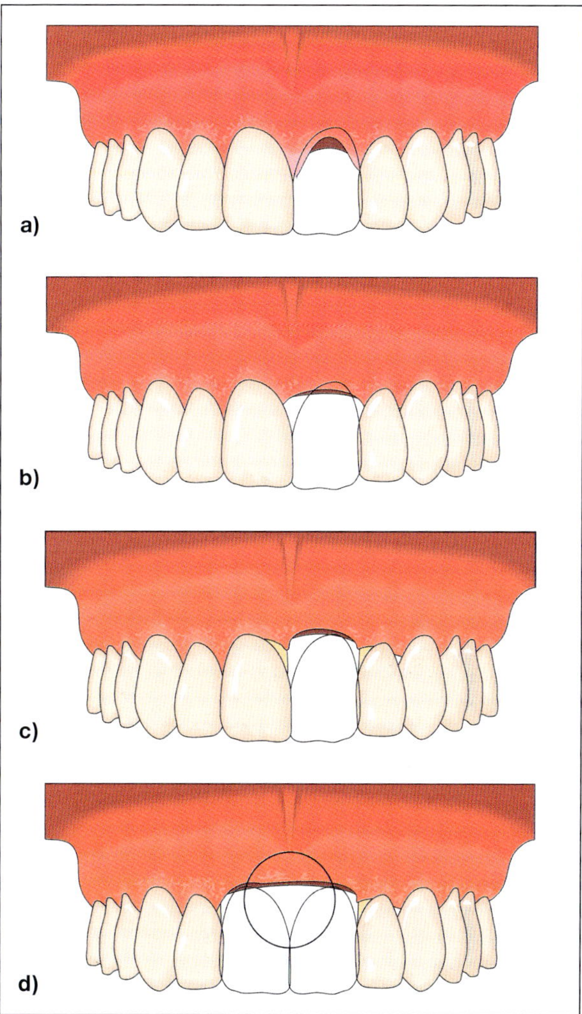

Fig 5-9 Vertical loss. **(a)** Class I: intact or slightly reduced papillæ. **(b)** Class II: limited loss of papillæ (less than 50% of papillæ loss). **(c)** Class III: severe loss of papillæ. **(d)** Class IV: absence of papillæ (edentulous ridge).

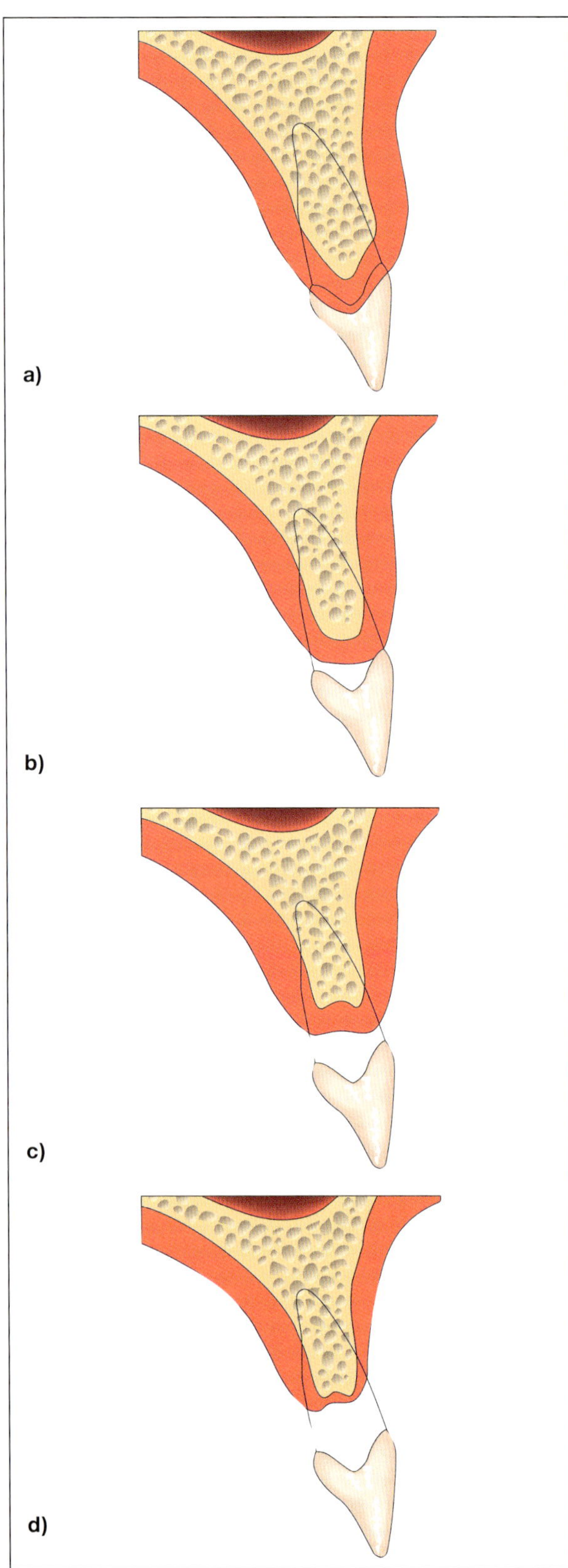

Fig 5-10 Horizontal loss. **(a)** Class A: intact or slightly reduced buccal tissue. **(b)** Class B: limited loss of buccal tissue. **(c)** Class C: severe loss of buccal tissue. **(d)** Class D: extreme loss of buccal tissue, often in combination with a limited amount of attached mucosa.

Horizontal loss (Fig 5-10)

Class A: intact or slightly reduced buccal tissue
Class B: limited loss of buccal tissue
Class C: severe loss of buccal tissue
Class D: extreme loss of buccal tissue, often in combination with a limited amount of attached mucosa.

Combinations of the different classes can exist according to each individual patient's situation. It is essential for the clinician to understand the complexity of the treatment and to be able to visualize the end result and understand its limitations.

Therefore, this classification should be used to document each anatomical situation before commencing treatment. It will guide the clinician in choosing proper treatment options to reach the expected final result.

It should be noted that the surgeon should respect the tissues and that a ridge augmentation should always be progressive, following the different steps of this classification.

Considering that each class is a step, the clinician should not expect to go directly from Class IV to Class II, or from Class III to Class I in one surgical procedure. A case can start in Class I and end up in Class I, or start in Class II and finish in Class I, but also start in Class IV and end up in Class III or II depending on the selected procedures or the treatment limitations. For example, when treating patients with an intact periodontal support or a limited ridge loss, the crown–abutment junction more or less coincides with the cemento-enamel junction of the neighboring teeth. In case of reduced periodontal support, where cemento-enamel junctions of the neighboring teeth are sub-marginally positioned and the base of the implant is at ridge level, the results will be a longer tooth, reduced or absent papillæ and esthetic problems in patients with a high lip line.

When dealing with esthetics, 4–5 mm in soft tissue height can dramatically change the final result, making each millimeter gained at each surgical step essential; for example:

- 2–3 mm in height can be gained using hard tissue augmentation procedures

- 2 mm can be gained using soft tissue augmentation procedures
- 1–2 mm can be gained using crown-lengthening techniques.

In total, these factors result in a 5–6 mm difference between different types of reconstruction concept. This 5–6 mm variation represents the difference between esthetic success and failure. This is why the clinician should carefully evaluate each patient before treatment using the NobelGuide concept. The clinical situation should be as close as possible to Class I to obtain an acceptable esthetic result. If not, the patient should accept a compromise esthetic situation or agree to undergo additive (hard and/or soft tissue) reconstructive surgeries.

During pre-surgical analysis, when assessing esthetics with the denture in place, several points should be taken into consideration:

- vertical dimension
- occlusion
- shape, color, positioning of the teeth
- lip support.

When trying the denture, the acrylic labial flange will give a certain amount of tissue support, which will disappear when the definitive implant-supported restoration is achieved. The most important point is the position of the new anterior teeth in relation with the lip and the labial portion of the teeth.

When dealing with the NobelGuide concept, the clinician should be aware of the different clinical options available:

- screw-retained restoration
- cemented restoration
- use of pre-fabricated abutments
- use of custom-made abutments
- definitive or temporary restorations.

In the presence of very high esthetic expectations, a temporary fixed restoration is preferable to a definitive Procera Implant Bridge.

During the following week, slight modifications of the peri-implant tissue may occur. The embrasures may be modified subsequently to control for hygiene, esthetics and phonetics. The patient may also need more time to become familiar with his or her new esthetics. Occlusion may also change during the following months.

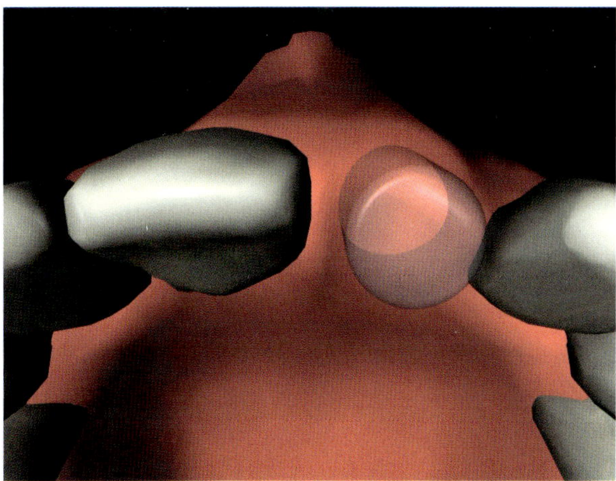

Fig 5-11 Occlusal view of a Class IA situation. The tissue-punch technique can be used here, assuming that hard and soft tissue quantities are sufficient. The cylinder represents the emergence profile of the abutment well integrated in the surrounding tissues.

In the presence of a lack of lip support or unfavorable esthetics, the teeth position, shape or size may need to be changed. The temporary restoration then becomes a base framework for the prosthondontist as well as for the patient, who can thus evaluate the necessity and the types of change to be performed.

Treatment planning

Figure 5-11 illustrates the different stages of ridge resorption. The tissue-punch technique can be used when facing an adequate ridge. As soon as the ridge resorbs, this technique will remove soft tissue instead of adding tissue. It is then apparent that another technique is needed to recreate optimal esthetics in this area (Fig 5-12).

A guideline for treatment options can be defined as follows.

- In the presence of Class IV or Class III loss where hard tissue reconstruction is required, all necessary surgeries needed to recreate the optimal ridge should be performed to maximize implant positioning.

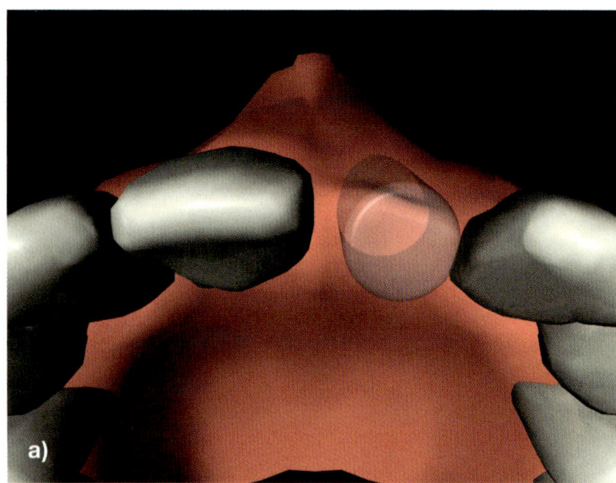

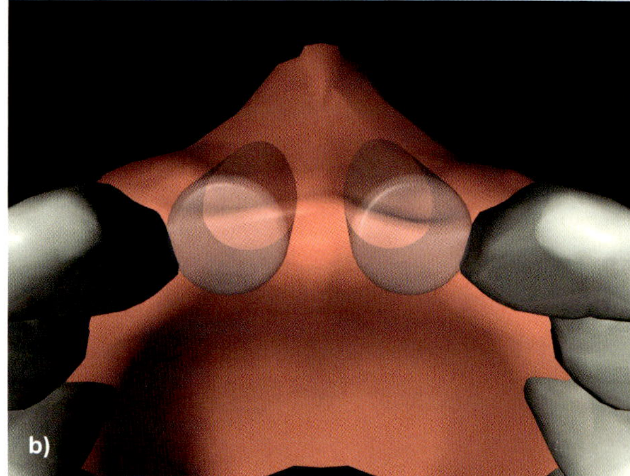

Fig 5-12 Due to ridge resorption and loss of tissue in the facial aspect, the abutment will emerge labially and apically, resulting in a compromised esthetic situation for single teeth **(a)** as well as multiple teeth **(b)**.

- In the presence of Class II loss, two options can be considered: (1) soft tissue augmentation before implant surgery, then use of flapless technique and removal of a certain amount of tissue with the counterbone when using the surgical guide before the drilling sequence; or (2) preserving all existing tissue by elevating a full-thickness flap and performing the papillæ regeneration technique (Palacci 2001). These two options use different approaches to get the same results. However, the clinician should consider the simplicity and reliability of the chosen technique. With the first option, additional surgeries have to be performed before implant placement. With the second option, a certain amount of existing soft tissue can be added vertically and horizontally to optimize papillæ reconstruction.

The use of the papillæ regeneration technique will help the clinician to gain tissues in these dimensions. However, a flap has to be elevated labially and the NobelGuide technique and concept have to be slightly modified. The labial flange has to be removed in the desired site, otherwise this will result in reduced stability of the surgical guide, loss of the horizontal anchored pins in this region and the need for an additive approach to retention of the guide.

During surgery, the clinician should always be sure of the optimal stability of the guide. In the case of a poor adaptation, a minor movement or a displacement of this guide will result in a improper implant position and inadequate prosthetic position with the following consequences:

- inadequate or poor fit
- poor contact points with the adjacent teeth
- poor occlusion with the opposite teeth
- eventual implant overload and loss of implants (as occlusion is a key factor for success in immediate loading)
- consequently, poor esthetics and an unsatisfied patient.

These surgeries will require extra time, effort and fees. Such issues need to be presented in detail to the patient.

Treatment options according to different classes

Class IVD

Fully edentulous patients

These patients can be treated successfully with the NobelGuide concept, if they present sufficient bone quantity and quality to be candidates for immediate loading. In those with inadequate bone quantity, the following surgeries can be performed prior to NobelGuide treatment to place enough

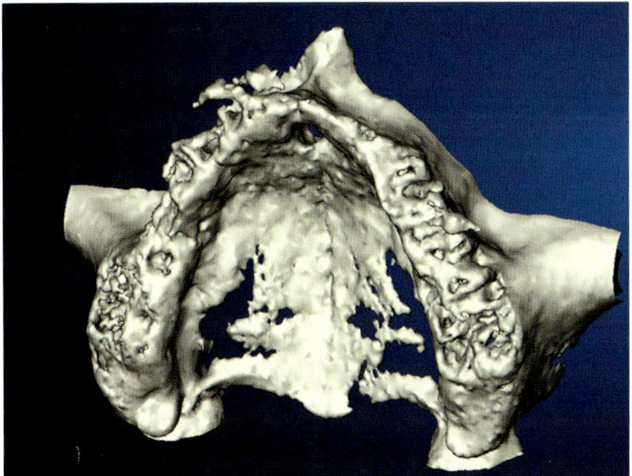

Fig 5-13 Three-dimensional reconstruction of an edentulous maxilla. Implant positioning will be determined by anatomical considerations: wide incisor canal, knife-edge ridge in anterior upper left quadrant, major bone loss in both cuspid positions and adequate bone quantity and quality in the premolar regions.

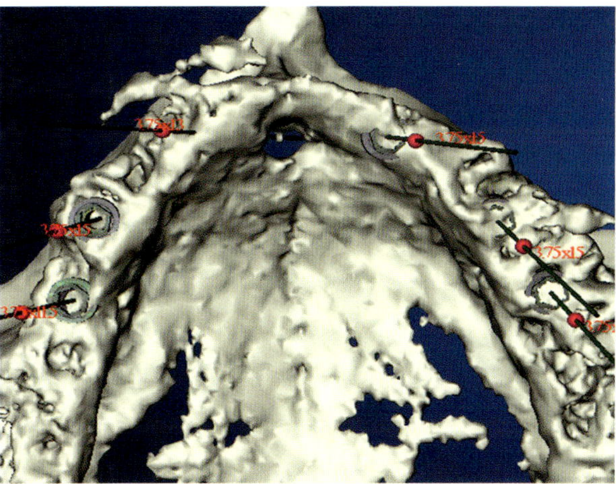

Fig 5-14 Implants will be placed in the lateral incisor regions and premolar regions to avoid anatomical structures, such as the incisor canal, and the severely resorbed ridges (e.g. the anterior maxilla and cuspid areas), which present severe defects.

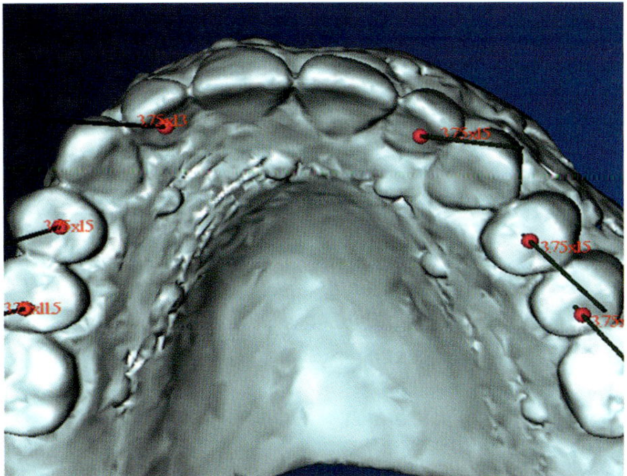

Fig 5-15 Placing the prosthetic restoration: implant positioning seems optimal in terms of emergence profile, stress distribution and hygiene and maintenance.

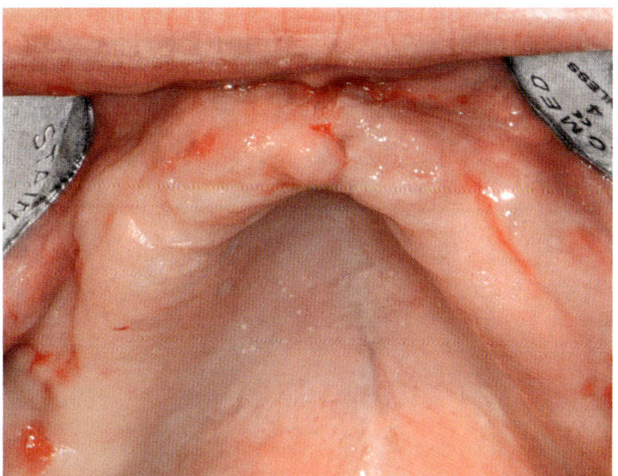

Fig 5-16 Clinical view of the edentulous maxilla.

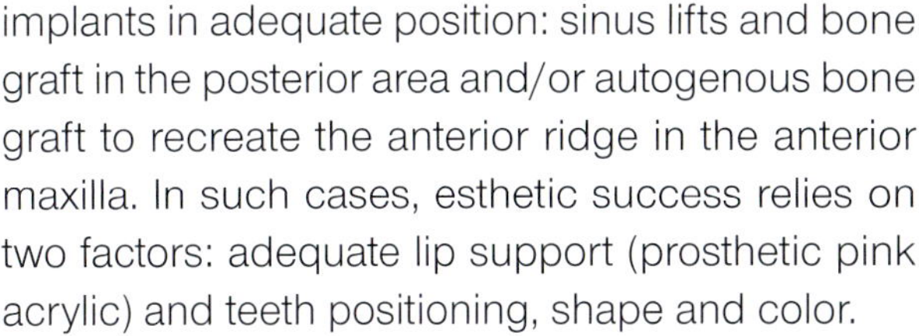

implants in adequate position: sinus lifts and bone graft in the posterior area and/or autogenous bone graft to recreate the anterior ridge in the anterior maxilla. In such cases, esthetic success relies on two factors: adequate lip support (prosthetic pink acrylic) and teeth positioning, shape and color.

The basic NobelGuide concept includes a presurgical guide based on an ideal denture set that is concordant with this treatment philosophy. The clinician will be able to finalize the future prosthesis and validate the teeth mounting shape, positioning and occlusion. Figs 5-13 to 5-19 illustrate the planning for a fully edentulous patient using the NobelGuide concept.

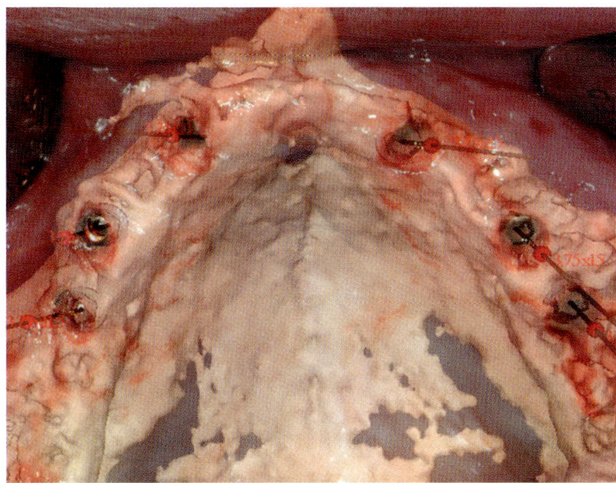

Fig 5-17 Superposition of the clinical view and virtual implant positioning.

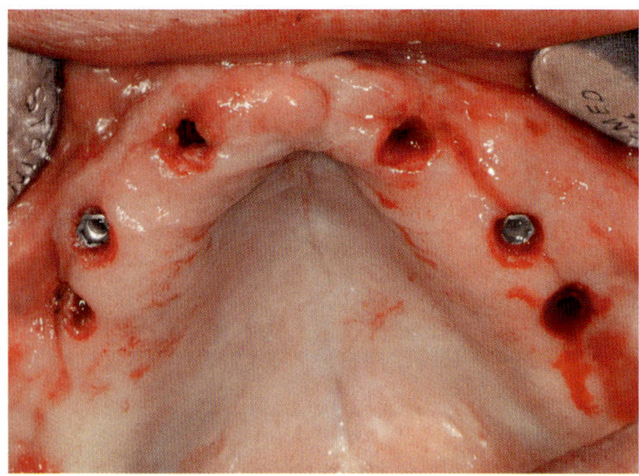

Fig 5-18 Correlation between computerized implant placement and the clinical situation after placing the implants.

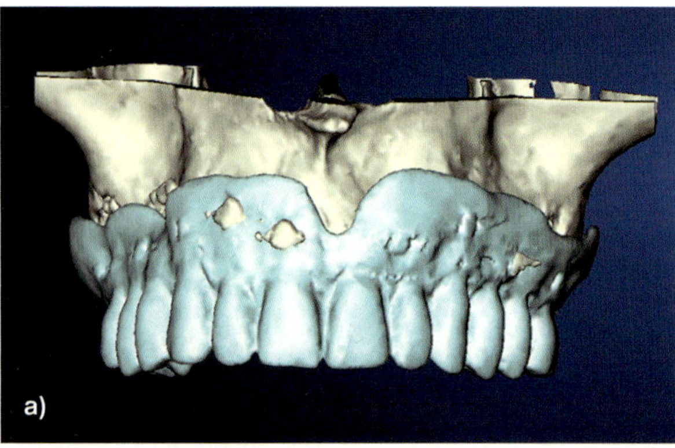

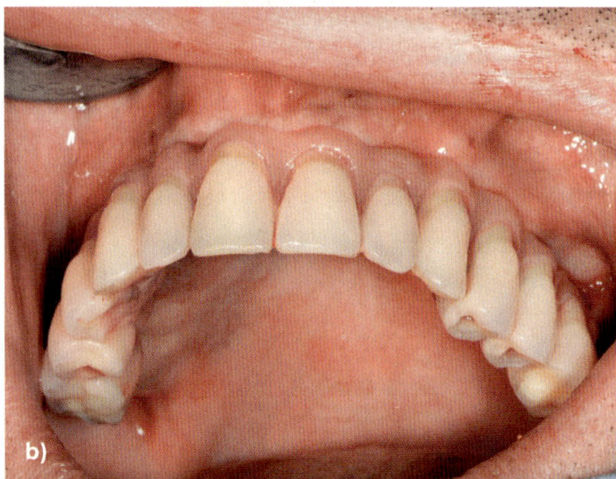

Figs 5-19 (a and b) Computerized and clinical views of the prosthetic restoration in place and the correlation between these two situations.

Partially edentulous patients

These patients can be treated in a similar way to the fully edentulous patient; however, esthetic expectations may be higher. Several problems can occur with this treatment, mainly due to the presence of teeth and limited available space to use the surgical guide and the extended drills, and to place implants.

The presence of teeth restricts the available space vertically and horizontally, i.e. vertically: tooth eruption, limited vertical dimension, and limited mouth opening; horizontally: bone resorption, teeth migration, and teeth angulation. If there is limited space, special attention should be given to placement of the guide cylinders into the acrylic guide. When analyzing the situation, radio opaque elements, such as crowns, posts and fillings, can produce scatters in the radiographic examinations. The clinician will then be unable to position the implants precisely using the Procera software, thus severely compromising the final result.

The radiological and surgical guide concept also has to be modified for these patients. The guide has to be perfectly adjusted to the existing teeth, otherwise incorrect implant placement will be faced, resulting in poor adjustment of the prosthesis on the implant; poor occlusion; unfavorable contact points, inducing food impaction; unfavorable hygiene; and/or deficient esthetics. To avoid these problems, windows should be opened against the occlusal surfaces of the teeth, allowing the fit control of the guide. Because of the presence of roots in dentate areas, stabilization pins can be impossible to place and should be replaced by clamps to stabilize the guide.

Figure 5-20 illustrates the planning of a partially edentulous patient using the NobelGuide concept.

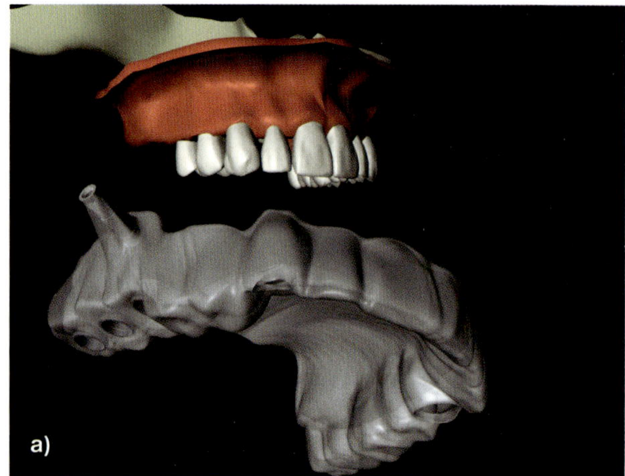

Fig 5-20 (a–p) Schematic drawings of the different steps for NobelGuide surgery on partially edentulous patient.

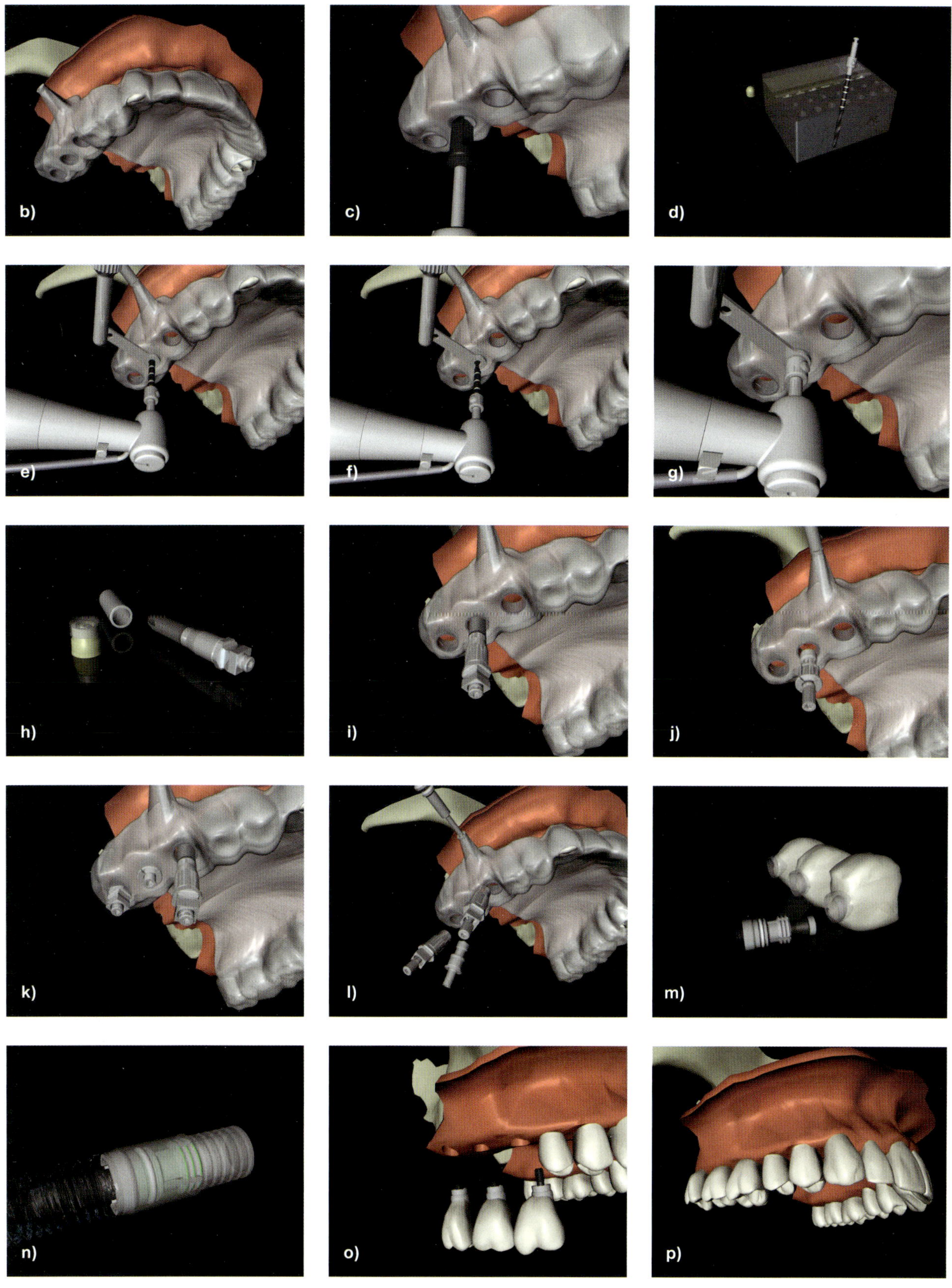
b)
c)
d)
e)
f)
g)
h)
i)
j)
k)
l)
m)
n)
o)
p)

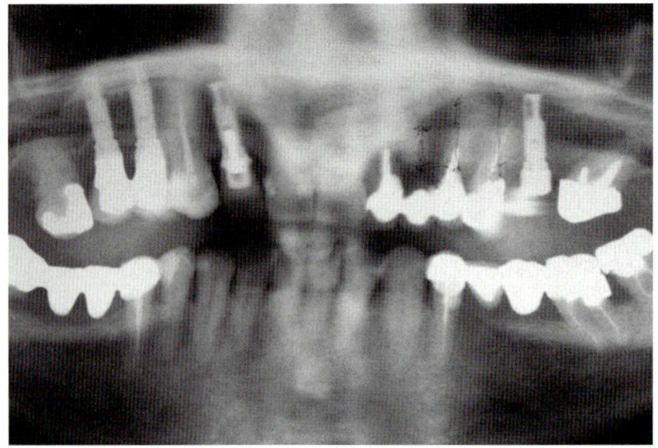

Fig 5-21 Panoramic radiograph of the patient in case 1.

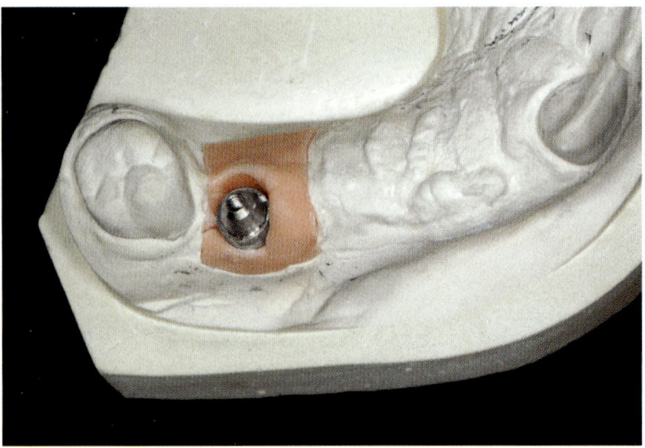

Fig 5-22 Clinical situation presented on the model including the abutment in place surrounded by pink soft acrylic.

Class IIIC

The NobelGuide concept will allow the clinician to optimize implant positioning into the existing bone providing that enough ridge is present. For patients with Class IIIC, hard tissue has to be added to the ridge to recreate adequate tissue support. In these situations, several treatment options can be chosen:

- bone grafting
- orthodontic eruption of the ridge
- osteogenesis distraction prior to implant placement.

If none of these options is appropriate, a porcelain/acrylic cosmetic element can be included in the final prosthesis to recreate acceptable lip support and achieve an esthetically successful result.

Class IIB and Class IA

In Class IIB and Class IA situations it is important to achieve a situation that is as close as possible to Class IA at the time of surgery. There are two possible scenarios: the patient is already in Class I, and the standard protocol is indicated in this situation; the patient is in Class II and additive soft tissue techniques are needed achieve Class I at implant installation.

Case presentations

Case I: precision of NobelGuide in some specific situation

In this patient, the existing fixed partial denture has to be removed and implants should be placed to restore function and esthetics. However, there are several problems in relation to the patient's need and the clinical situation. The patient would like to avoid wearing a removable temporary restoration and an impacted canine is present. The clinician should avoid extracting this tooth because of the major defect that would result from this extraction (Fig 5-21).

Knowing that a fixed temporary restoration should be placed immediately after implant insertion, an implant was placed in the site of the first maxillary molar. A 6-month healing time was observed for osseointegration and to minimize the load on future anterior implants (limited in length owing to the position of the impacted canine) (Fig 5-22).

By using the NobelGuide concept with Procera software, the clinician can evaluate possible positioning of two implants in the edentulous zone (Fig 5-23). The three-dimensional analysis confirms the possibility of placing an 8.5 mm implant above (see Fig 5-31) the impacted tooth and an 11.5 mm implant more distally.

A fixed temporary restoration can then be planned, providing that the distal implant will be integrated into the prosthetic restoration and that

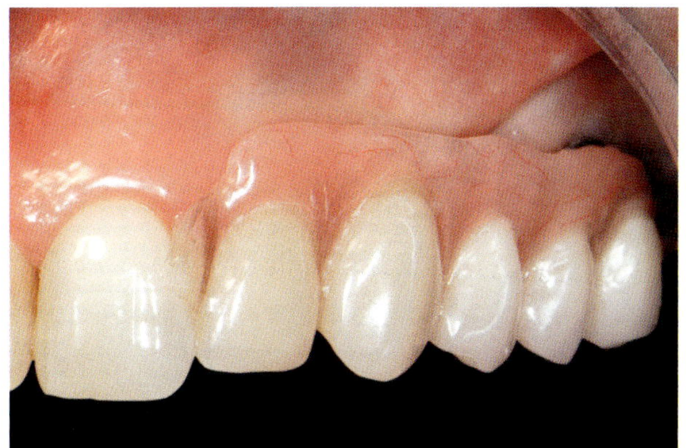

Fig 5-23 Prosthetic guide in place allowing evaluation of the clinical, surgical and prosthetic options. The labial flange in the upper left lateral and cuspid position indicates that some surgical manipulations are needed to optimize the final esthetic result.

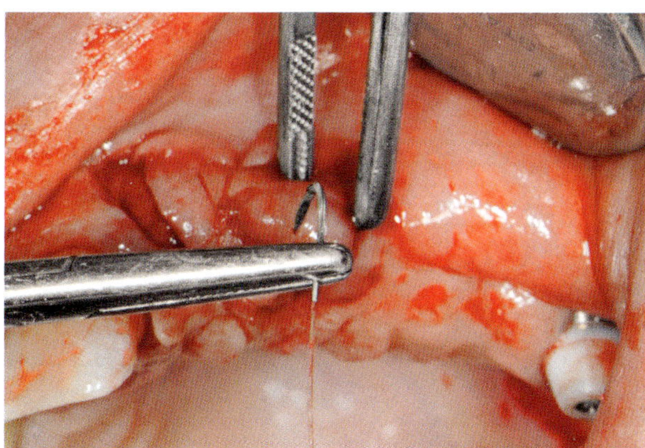

Fig 5-25 A connective tissue graft is harvested in the intraoral cavity and sutured on to the internal side of the flap to maximize ridge augmentation in the desired position.

all the mesial portion of the fixed partial denture will be out of occlusion.

In terms of esthetic considerations, the patient has moderate lip mobility as well as a reasonably high lip line. However, the clinician should focus on the esthetics of the more anterior portion of this restoration, i.e. the emergence profile of the lateral incisor and the canine.

A connective tissue graft, harvested in the palatal area, was performed, allowing a more adequate ridge contour prior to implant placement. This graft was placed into the internal side of the flap and sutured into position, as shown in the schematic illustration (Fig 5-24).

A full-thickness flap was elevated and releasing incisions were made to give flexibility to the flap. A connective tissue graft was harvested in the tuberosity area and de-epithelialized, then sutured into the desired position. The graft can be placed more or less coronally according to the esthetic needs. The flap is then sutured (Figs 5-25 and 5-26).

After 4 weeks, the texture, shape and color of

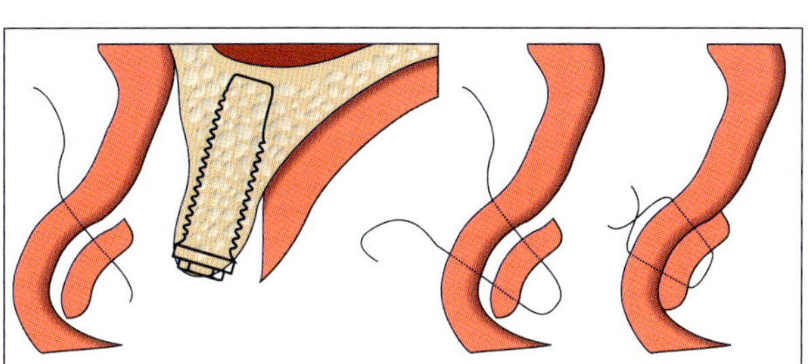

Fig 5-24 Schematic drawing illustrating the positioning of the graft in the internal side of the flap.

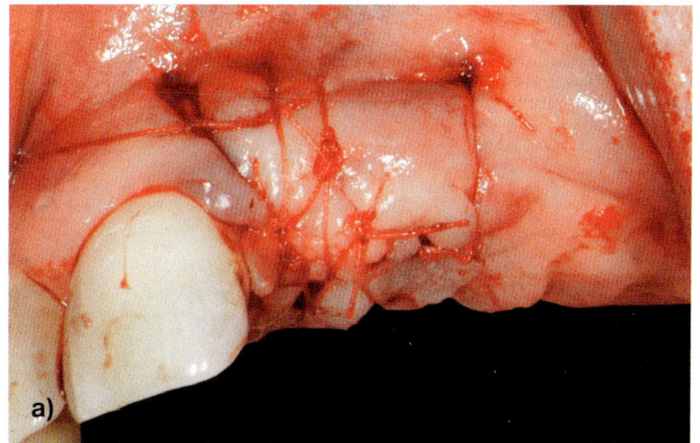

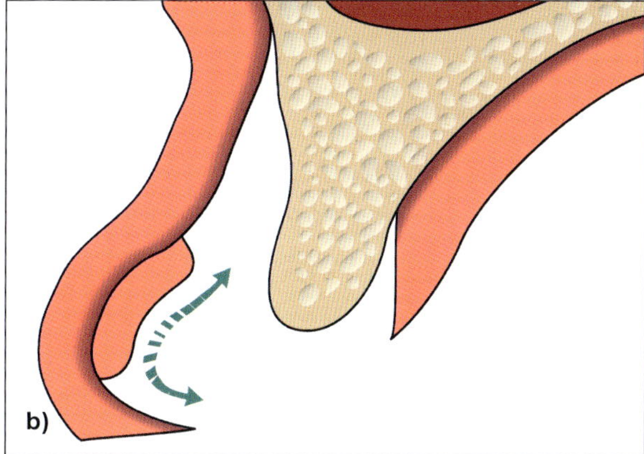

Fig 5-26 Clinical **(a)** and schematic **(b)** view of the sutured graft.

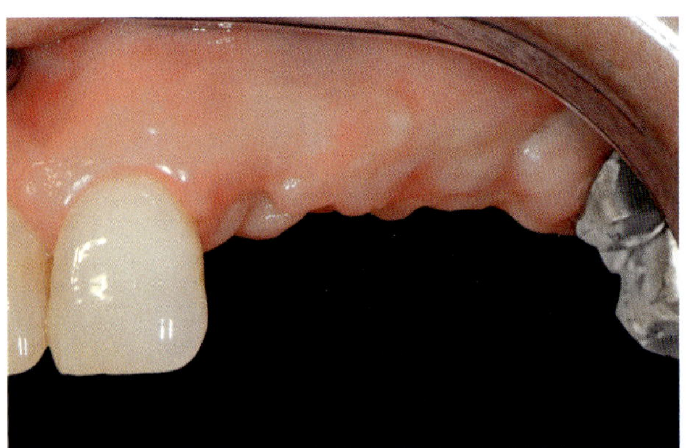

Fig 5-27 Clinical result of the ridge augmentation 2 months after mucogingival surgery. Guided surgery can then be planned.

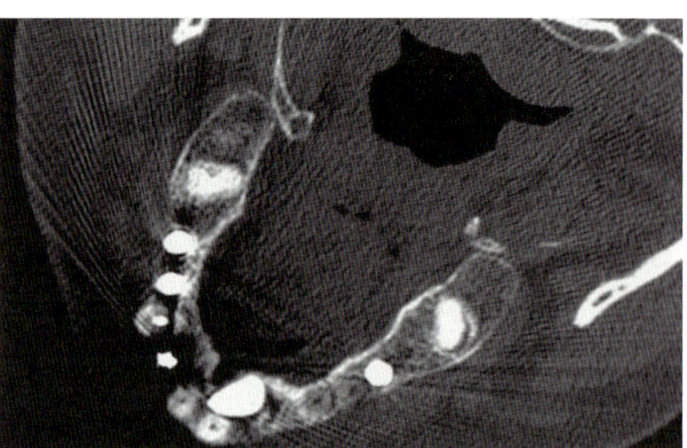

Fig 5-29 Occlusal cut illustrating the position of the impacted cuspid and the implant.

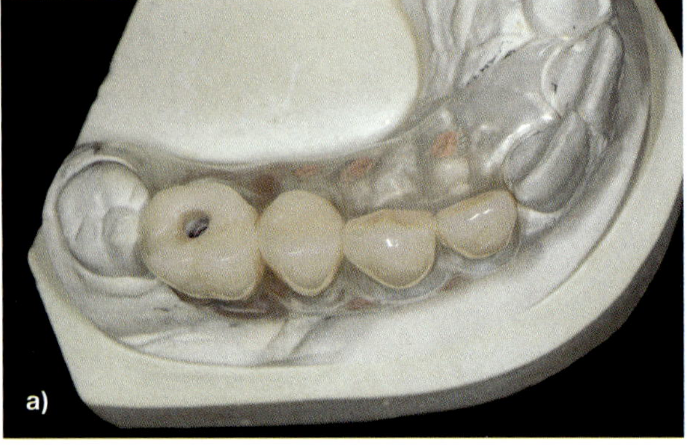

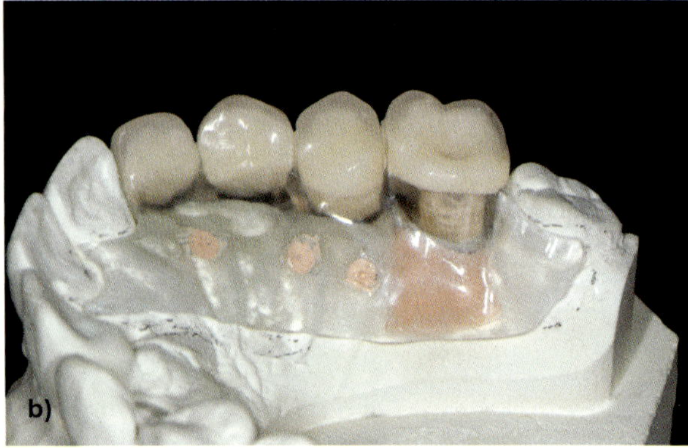

Fig 5-28 Prosthetic guide including gutta-percha markers in place: **(a)** labial and **(b)** palatal views. Note the position of the markers in different planes and the labial flange.

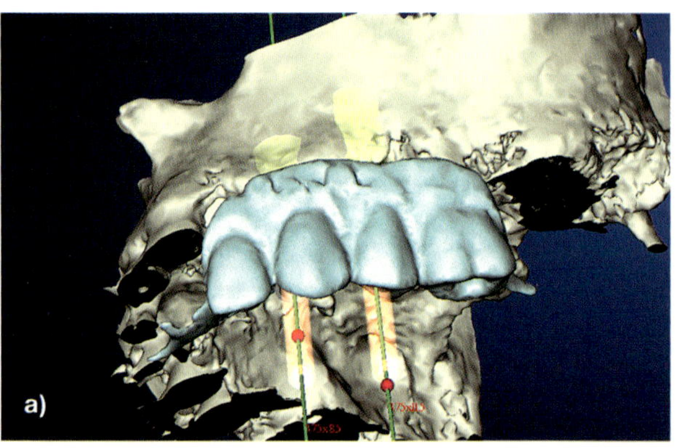

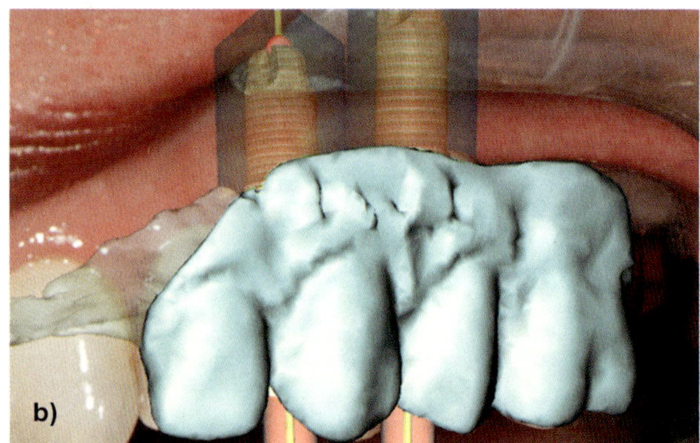

Fig 5-30 (a and b) Three-dimensional reconstruction with the guide in place. Implant placement is optimized in accordance with the anatomic structures, limitations and the future prosthetic restoration.

the soft tissue are optimal (Fig 5-27). A radiological guide is fabricated with acrylic teeth, and gutta-percha markers are placed labially and palatally according to the protocol. The guide is stabilized by the existing implant (Fig 5-28).

A significant difference can be seen between the clinical situation at the first surgical evaluation, using the esthetic model with pink acrylic in the labial zone, and the surgical situation after healing of the graft (Fig 5-22).

Using a double impression technique, the existing implant will be used to stabilize the radiologic stent as well as the surgical guide (Fig 5-28).

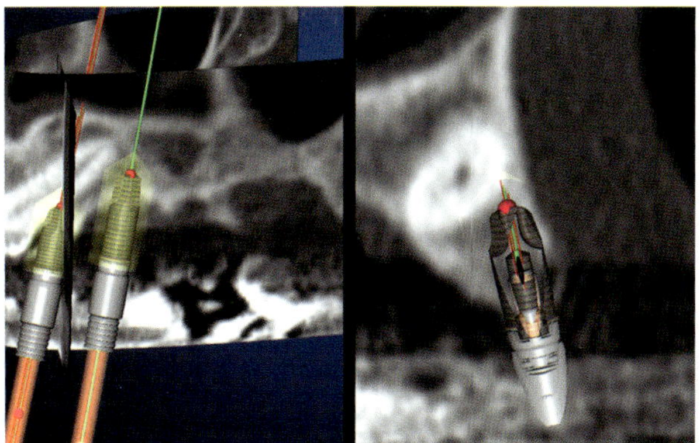

Fig 5-31 Precision in implant positioning above the impacted canine.

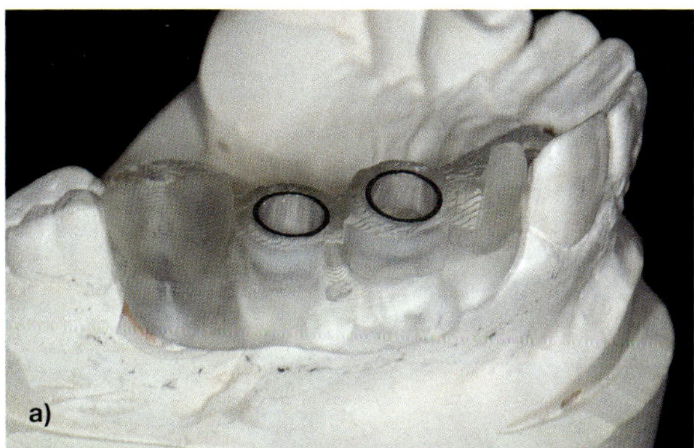

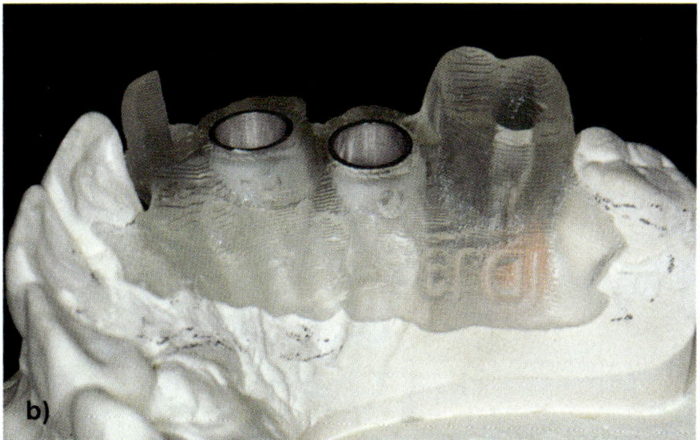

Fig 5-32 The surgical guide is fabricated and positioned on the model; the distal implant will be used to stabilize this guide. **(a)** Labial and **(b)** palatal view.

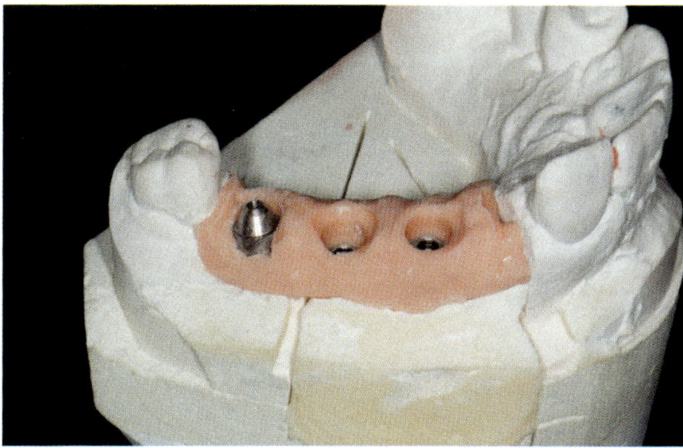

Fig 5-33 The model is fabricated: the implant replicas are fixed into the copings and the soft acrylic material and stone are poured on top.

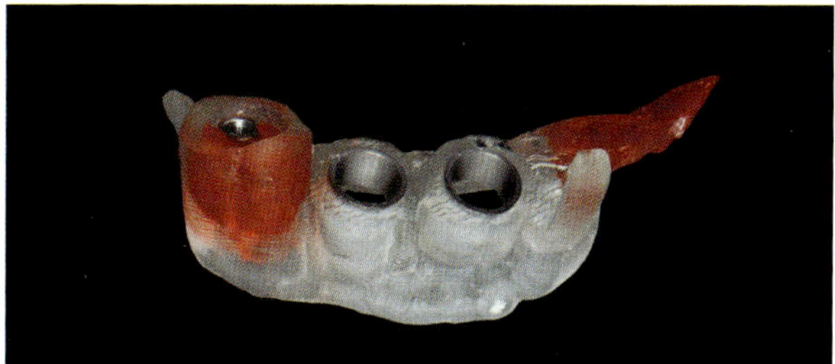

Fig 5-34 The surgical guide is modified to achieve stabilization. A gold cylinder is included distally above the implant already in place, and an acrylic extension will stabilize the guide mesially. No guide pins can be placed because of tthe impacted tooth.

Before surgery, the passive fit of the guide has to be carefully checked. This guide is then screw retained to the multi-unit abutment at the time of the surgery, allowing the precise positioning of the two implants. The temporary restoration is then screwed into position through adjustable abutments.

The passive fit of the prosthesis, the emergence profile and occlusion are controlled. After 4 months, the definitive restoration is placed using a multi-unit abutment.

In this case, the use of the NobelGuide concept has assisted the clinician to visualize the impacted canine and place the implants with a precise technique without reflecting any flap. It has enabled calculation of the implant position and length to optimize implant positioning in the overall concept.

Use of the NobelGuide concept also allows for the possibility of going through to a fixed immediate temporary restoration, and to combine the use of an existing implant with the newly placed implants (Figs 5-29 to 5-37).

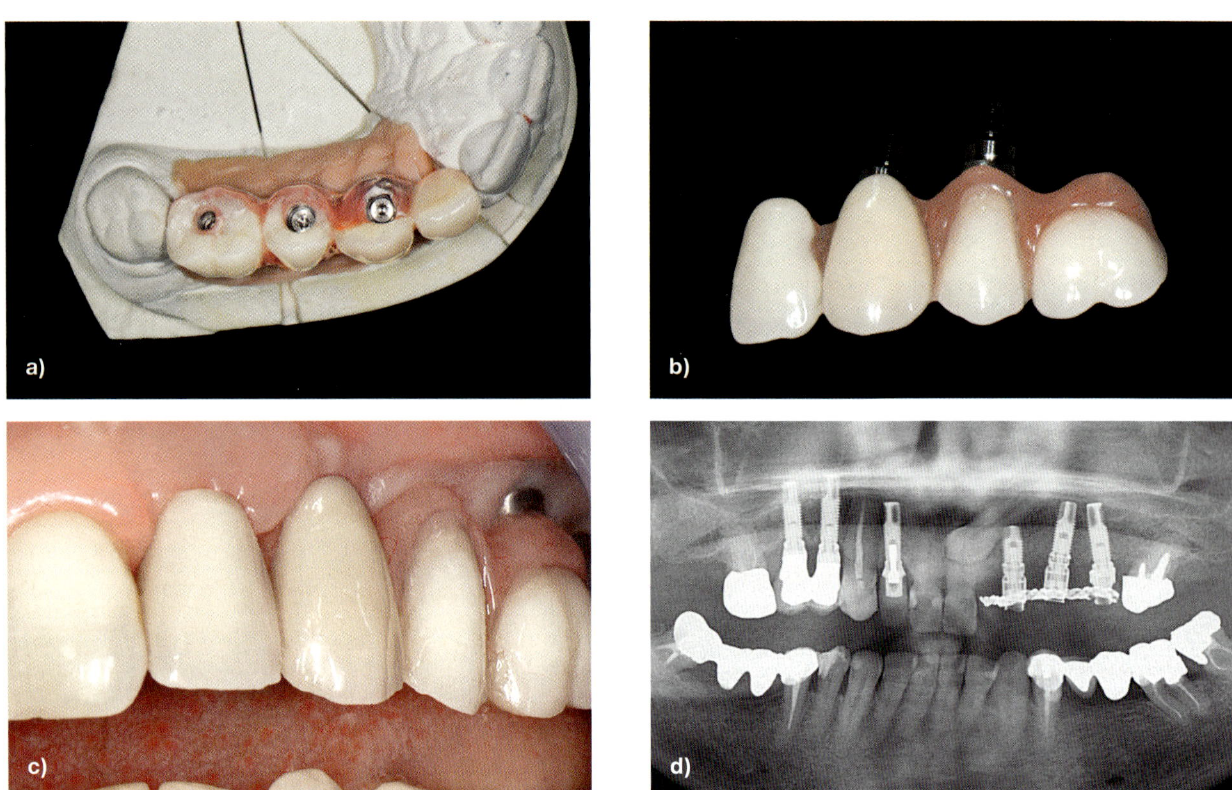

Fig 5-35 (a and b) Temporary prosthetic restoration. (c) At 4 days post-operation. (d) Radiograph illustrating the perfect correspondence between the analysis and the clinical situation.

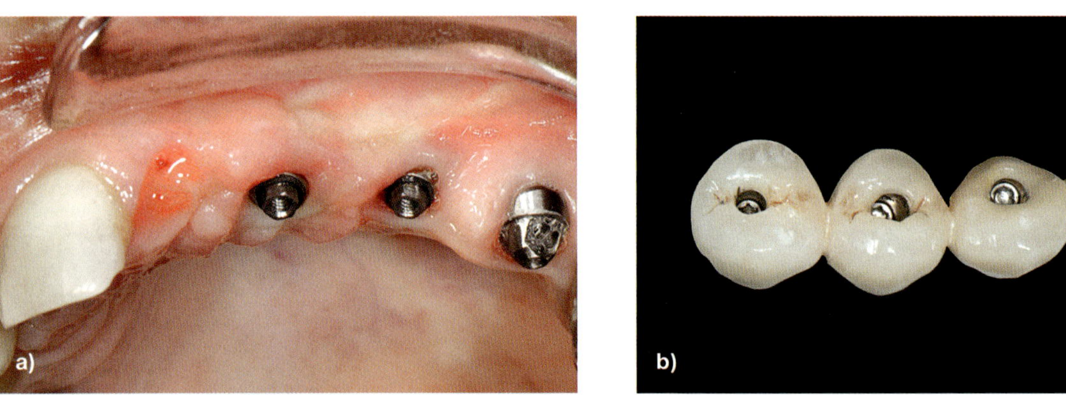

Fig 5-36 (a and b) Six months later, abutments are changed to a multi-unit abutment and a porcelain-fused-to-metal reconstruction is fabricated.

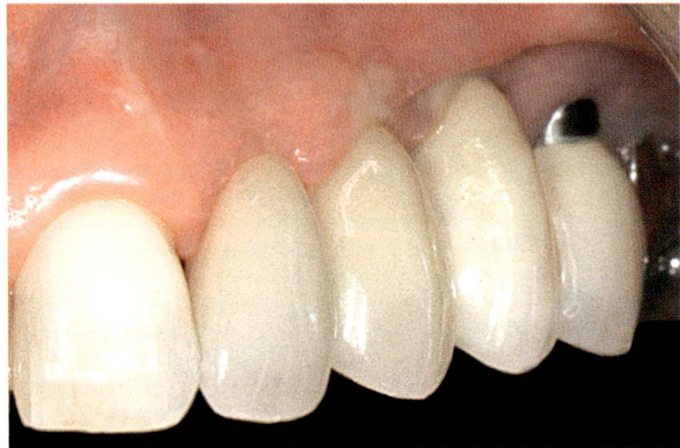

Fig 5-37 Clinical situation 6 months after implant surgery.

Case II: combinations of extractions and implant placement using NobelGuide

Some specific clinical situations may be problematic when using the NobelGuide system. For example, where certain teeth or roots need to be extracted, immediate implant placement can be compromised by the difficulty of correctly placing the implants in the alveolæ in the software and intraorally and the possible lack of stability of the placed implants. Also, the existing teeth, crowns and roots to be extracted may interfere with correct adaptation of the guide.

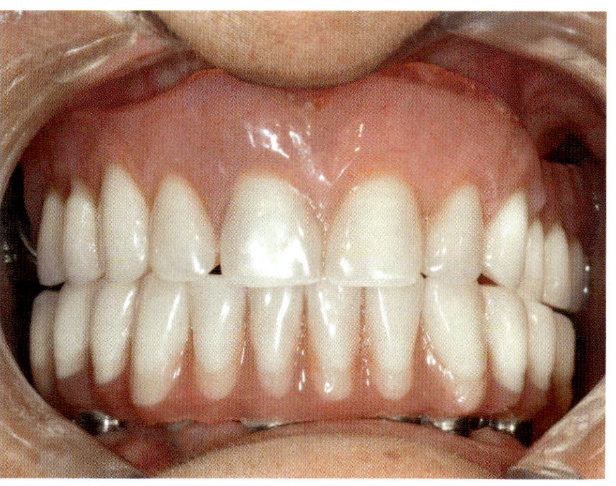

Fig 5-38 Clinical situation: fixed anchored partial denture in the mandible, removable denture in the maxilla.

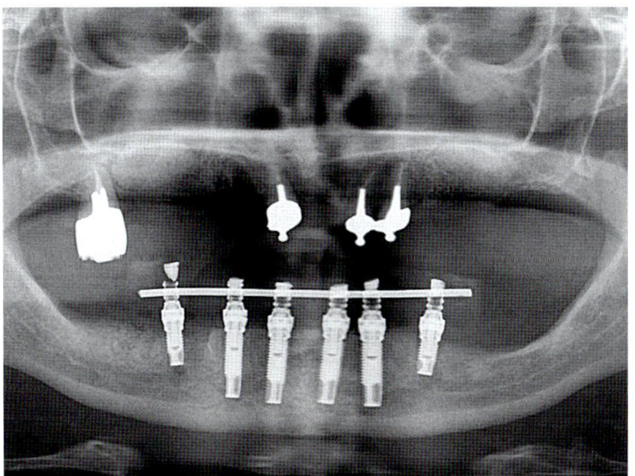

Fig 5-39 Panoramic radiograph showing bone grafts in the posterior areas, and teeth to be extracted in the front.

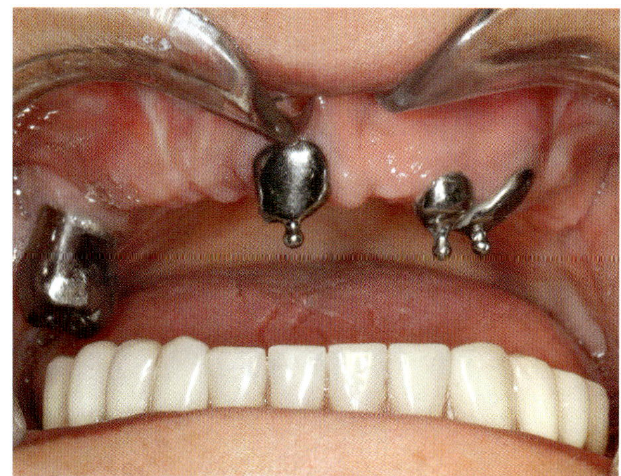

Fig 5-40 Molar and anterior teeth supporting the attachments have to be extracted.

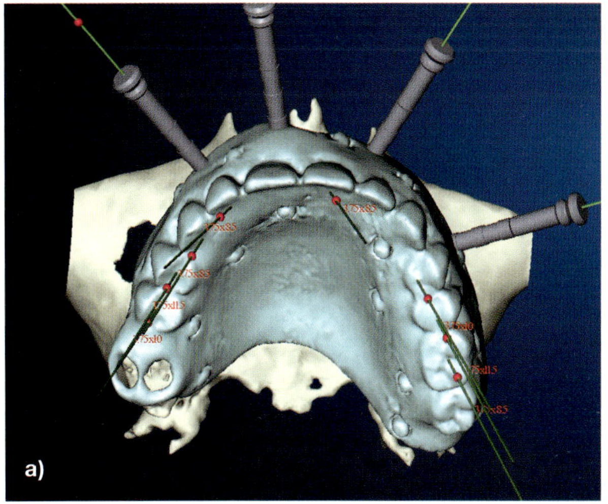

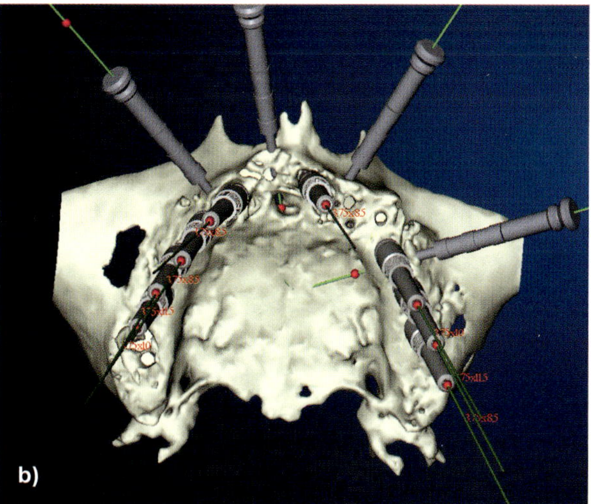

Fig 5-41 (a and b) Placement of the implants removing the existing roots as shown on Procera software.

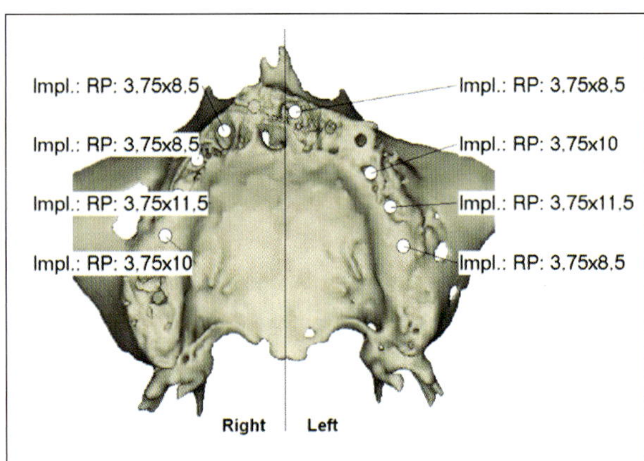

Fig 5-42 Schematic drawing illustrating position and length of the implants.

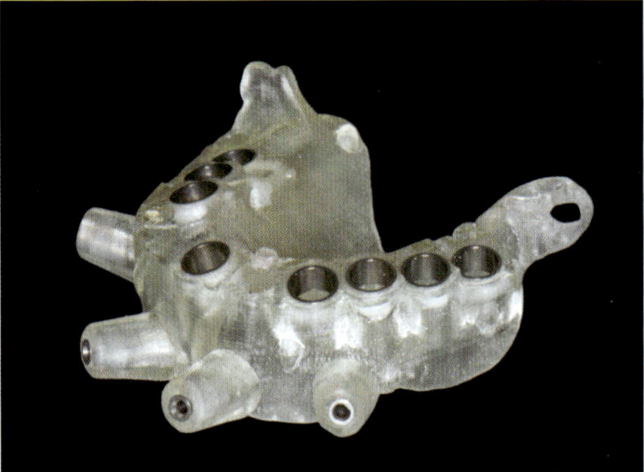

Fig 5-43 Only the six posterior implants will be placed using the surgical guide. The anterior sleeves are used for placing replicas on the model.

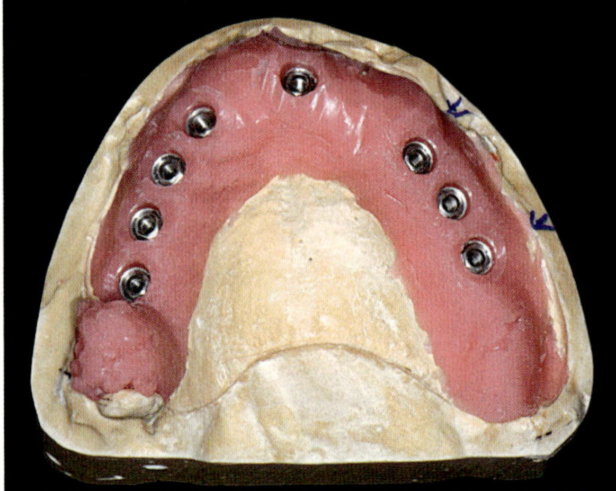

Fig 5-44 Model with soft acrylic material. Four multi-unit abutments will be placed on the two distal and intermediate implants.

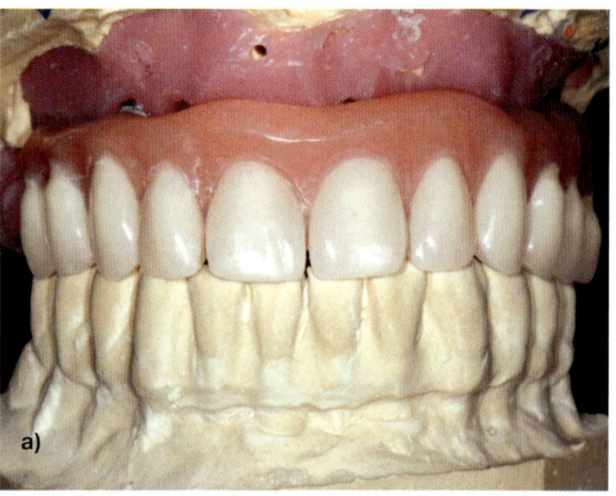

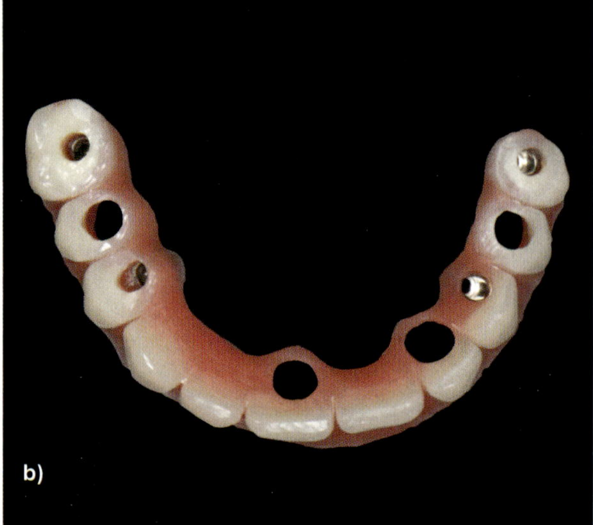

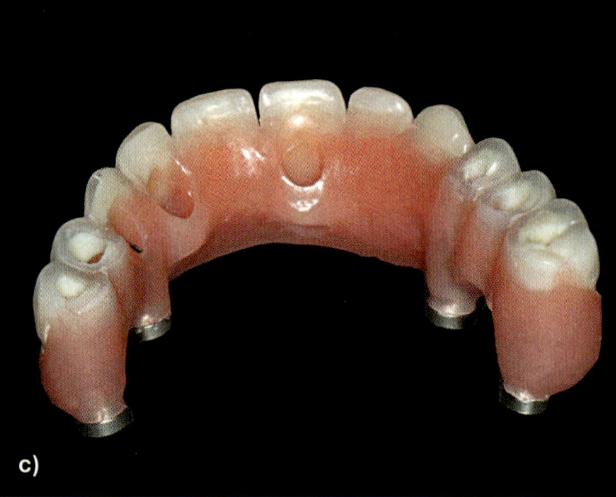

Fig 5-45 (a–c) Temporary prosthetic restoration on the articulator and different views of the fixed partial denture (occlusal, palatal). Holes where the restoration will be connected by acrylic material to the abutment allow for a precise fit.

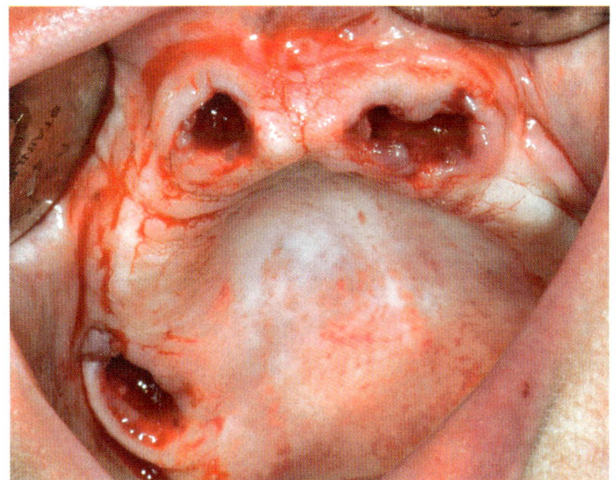

Fig 5-46 Extraction of the roots, allowing placement of the guide.

A clinical evaluation may be required to assess areas to be treated. A possible solution is the combined use of the guide, the temporary fixed partial denture and a more conventional implant treatment. The following case report illustrates this treatment option.

The patient, a 58-year-old female who had already benefited from a fixed implant restoration in the mandible, was willing to undergo the same type of treatment in the maxilla. The removable existing restoration was no longer satisfactory for her, and the roots supporting precision attachments had to be extracted (Figs 5-38 to 5-40).

The maxilla was prepared when placing the implants in the mandible by adding hard tissue in the posterior maxilla areas using a sinus elevation and bone grafting technique. Six months' later, the conventional protocol was applied and five implants were positioned in the maxilla using Procera software (Figs 5-41 to 5-53).

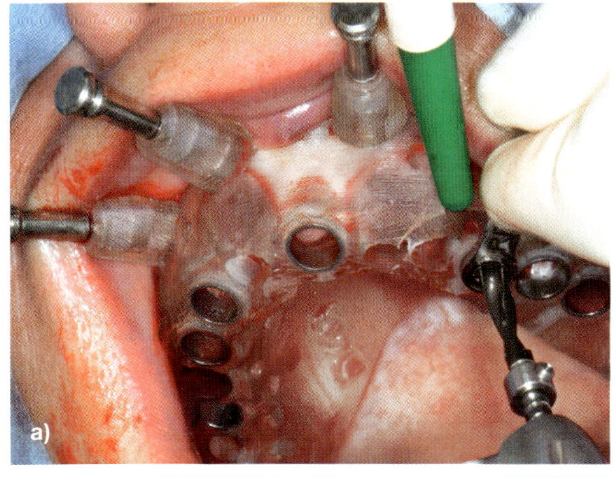

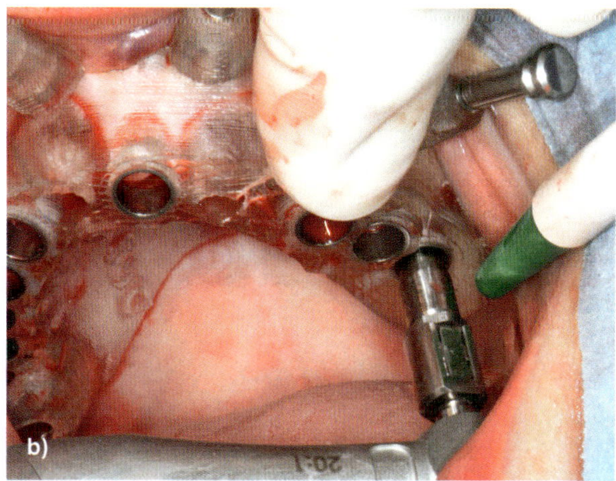

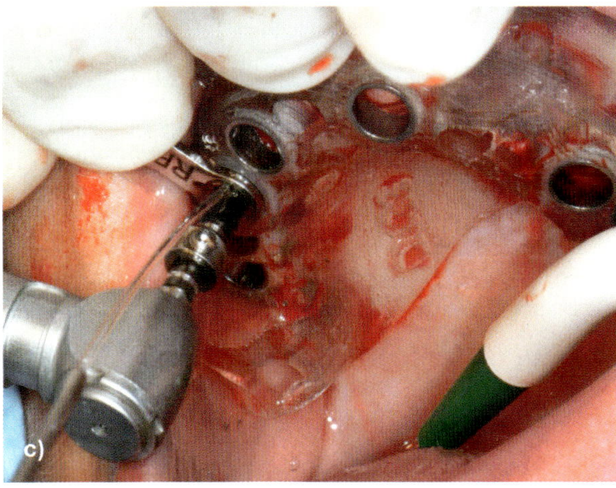

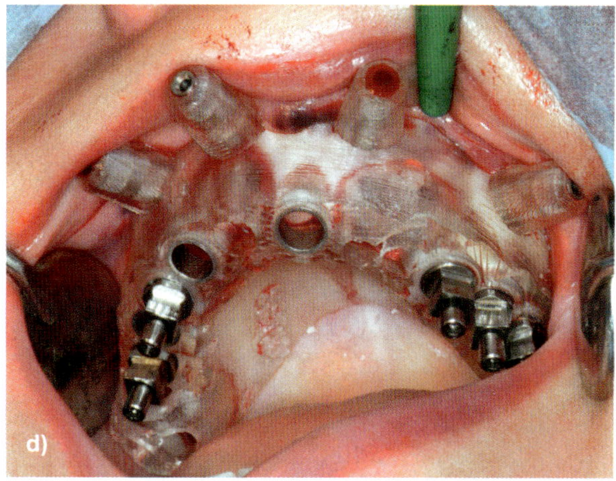

Fig 5-47 (a–d) Placement of the six posterior implants according to the protocol.

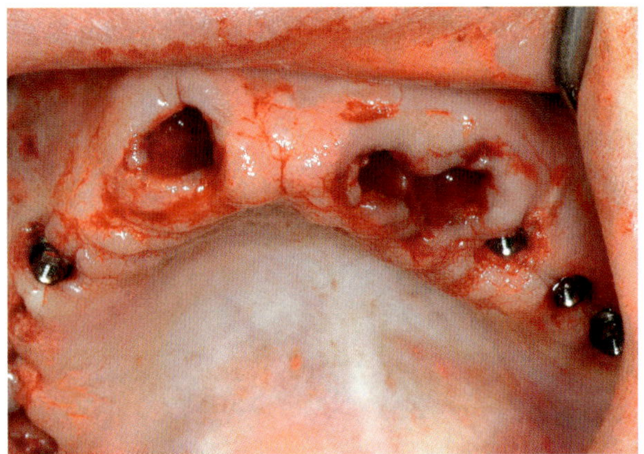

Fig 5-48 The guide is then removed, bone spicules around implants are eliminated using a trefine, and the multi-unit abutment is screwed onto the six implants.

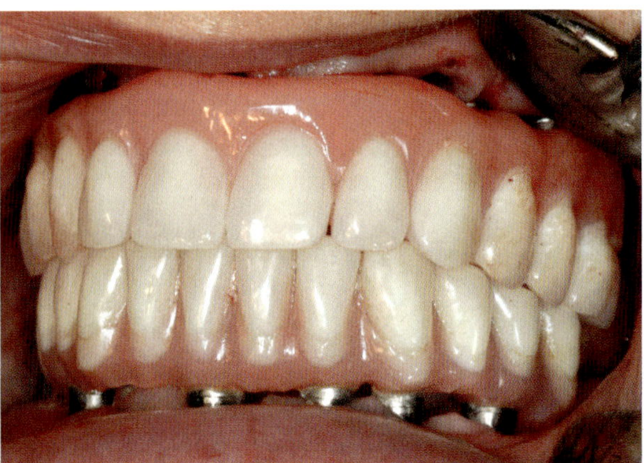

Fig 5-49 The fixed partial denture is placed, and position and occlusion are checked. A drill will go through the anterior holes to locate the position of the more anterior fixtures. The fixed partial denture is then removed.

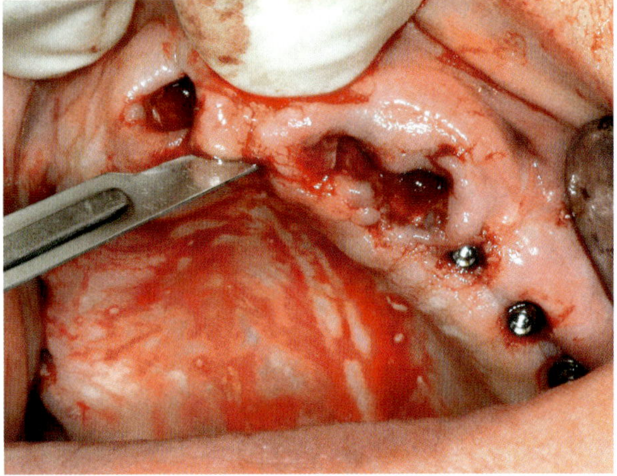

Fig 5-50 A flap is elevated. Implants are placed according to the pre-determined position, but there is an option to choose the optimal position according to the clinical situation (shape of the ridge, defects, bone quality).

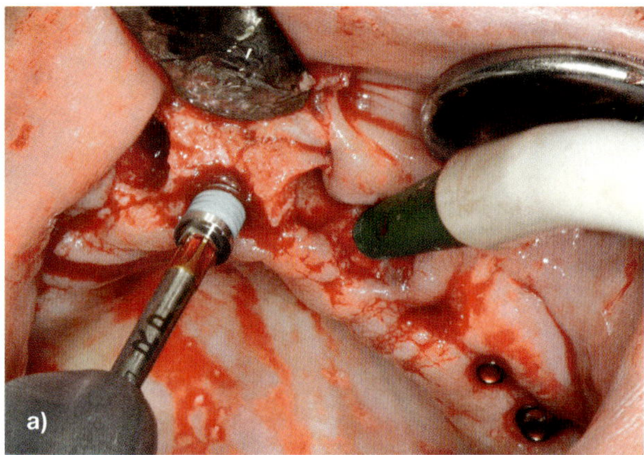

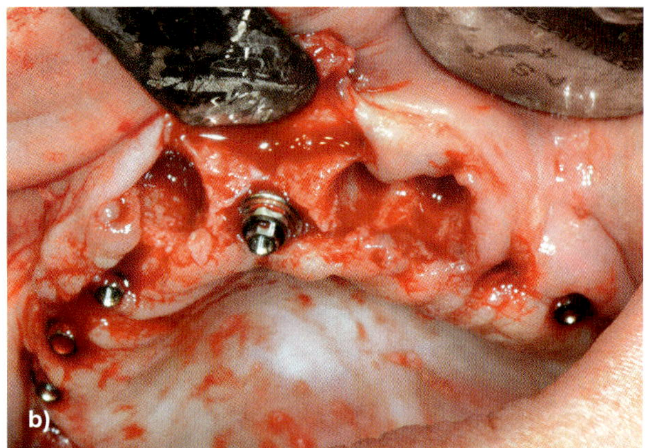

Fig 5-51 (a and b) Implants are inserted and abutments placed.

A surgical guide was then fabricated, but only six of the eight implants were placed using this guide: the two anterior implants were placed without use of the guide. The prosthetic restoration was fabricated, but only four titanium cylinders were connected on the multi-unit abutments placed on the model. This allowed use of multi-unit abutments for all the prosthetic restoration.

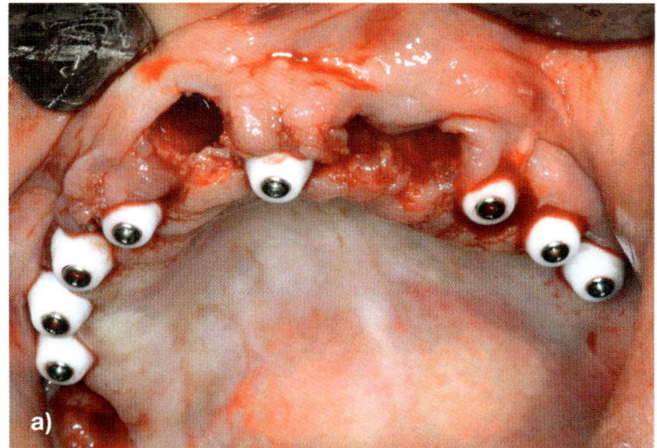

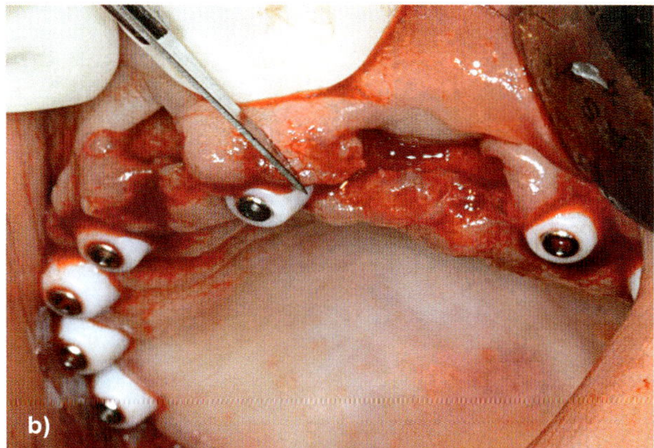

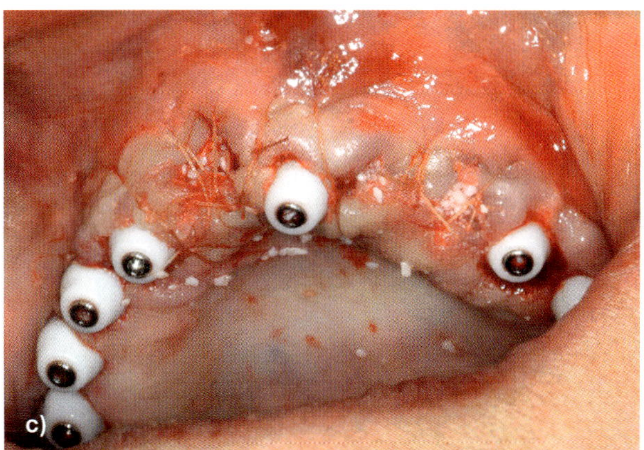

Fig 5-52 (a–c) The alveolæ previously cleaned are filled with allogenic material to prevent future resorption. Soft tissue is manipulated to optimize closure of the flap and its adaptation around the abutments.

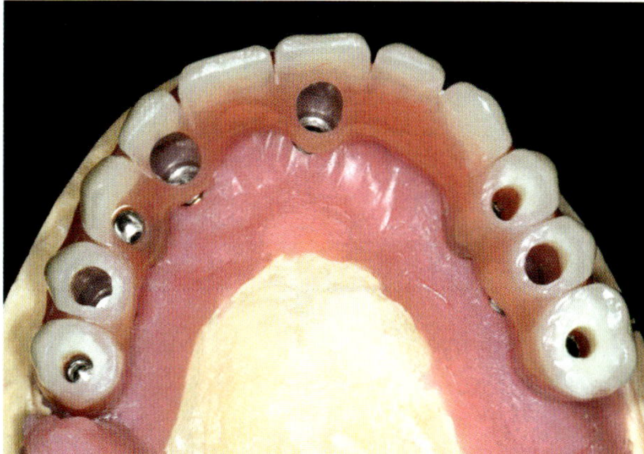

Fig 5-53 (a) The connection of the fixed partial denture to the implants is made. This connection can be done either intraorally, by inserting acrylic material between the titanium cylinders screwed and the abutments and the prosthetics, or in the laboratory by taking an impression of the abutments. In both cases, chair time will be significantly reduced compared with a more conventional protocol, adding comfort to the patient and the prosthodondist.

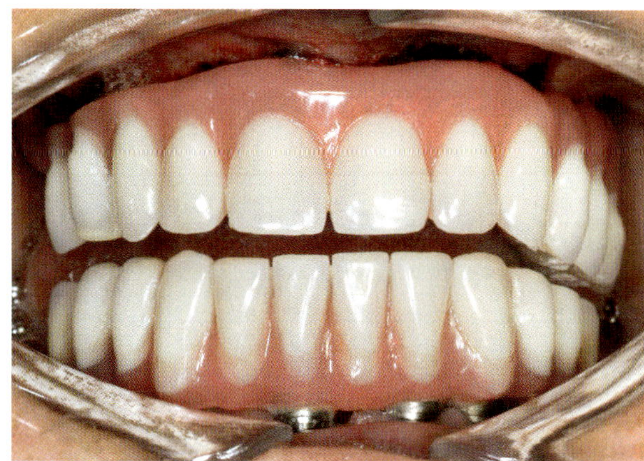

Fig 5-53 (b) View of the temporary restoration in place 24 hours after surgery (prosthodontist: Dr Christian Richelme, Marseille).

The objective is to construct the fixed partial denture, find its precise position, achieve optimal esthetics and occlusion, and connect this fixed partial denture to the remaining implants and abutments when seated on four implants. This allows application of the basic NobelGuide concept, optimizes the fit of the prosthetic restoration as well as occlusion, and limits prosthetic manipulations .

Clinical time is reduced in comparison with the conventional protocol. The prosthodontist will only have to connect the abutments to the restoration by adding resin into the holes in regard to the implants sites. The benefits for the clinicians and the patient are evident. This very reliable technique can be applied in various situations, thus adding more flexibility to the original concept.

Case III: soft tissue manipulation – papillæ regeneration technique

A 53-year-old female patient presented with loss of four maxillary incisors and maxillary right cuspid following trauma. After a healing period, the Nobel-Guide treatment option was presented to her. Clinical examination and esthetic and occlusal analyses on models was undertaken. Radiological examination showed the possibility of placing three implants (two of 15 mm and one of 13 mm), allowing the placement of a five-unit temporary fixed partial denture (Figs 5-54 to 5-56).

However, if the hard tissue anatomy was sufficient to allow the placement of three implants, the soft tissue contour was such that a tissue-punch technique would jeopardize the final esthetic result. It was then decided to reflect a full-thickness flap in the buccal direction to save as much tissue as possible (Fig 5-57).

After placement of the three implants using the surgical guide (Figs 5-58 to 5-60), the papillæ regeneration technique was used in combination with a connective tissue graft to recreate the papillæ and to reconstruct the ridge where too much tissue was lost (Figs 5-60 and 5-61). A temporary fixed partial denture was then placed on the 2 mm multi-unit abutment. This enabled immediate function and esthetics for this patient (Figs 5-62 and 5-63).

Four months later, the definitive porcelain-fused-to-metal fixed partial denture was fabricated. When removing the temporary fixed partial denture, the quality, quantity, texture and color of the peri-implant soft tissue were found to be satisfactory (Figs 5-64 to 5-67).

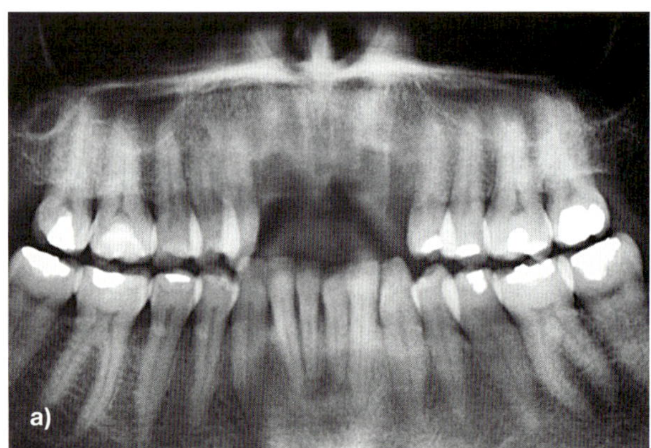

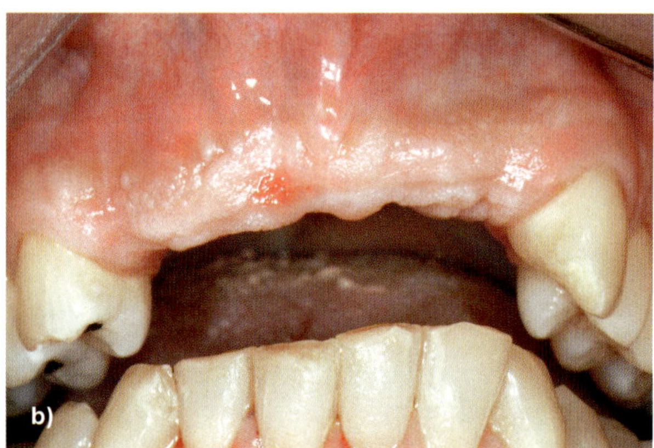

Fig 5-54 (a) Panoramic radiograph. **(b)** Clinical situation: some horizontal bone loss, as well as vertical bone loss, can be seen. The papillæ have disappeared.

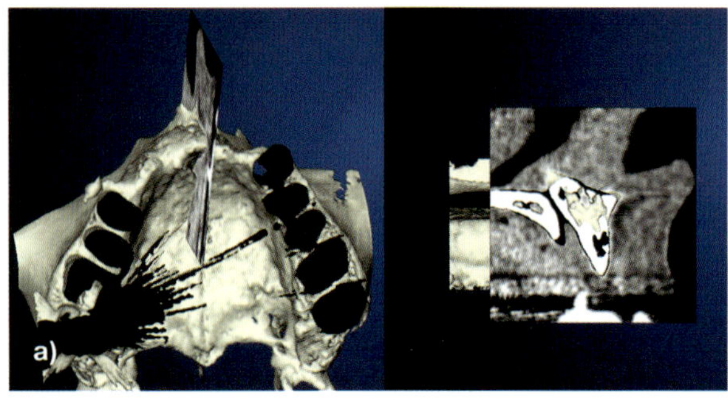

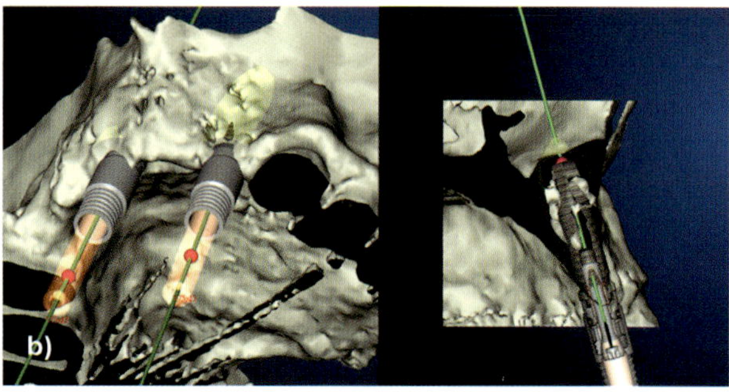

Fig 5-55 (a and b) Occlusal view on Procera software shows the importance of the incisor canal and the thin ridge in the anterior segment.

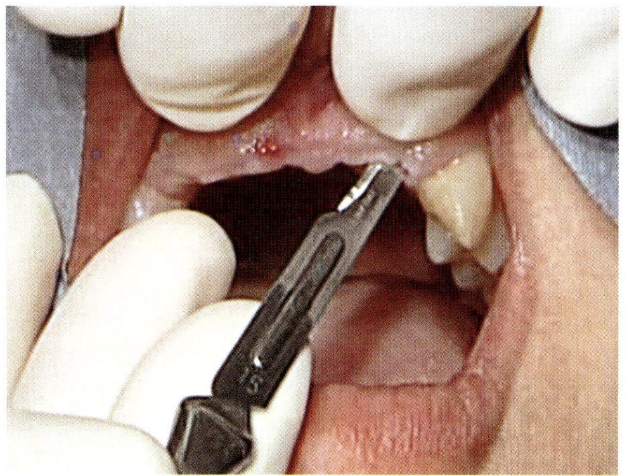

Fig 5-56 Optimal implant and abutment placement. A horizontal incision is made, slightly palatal.

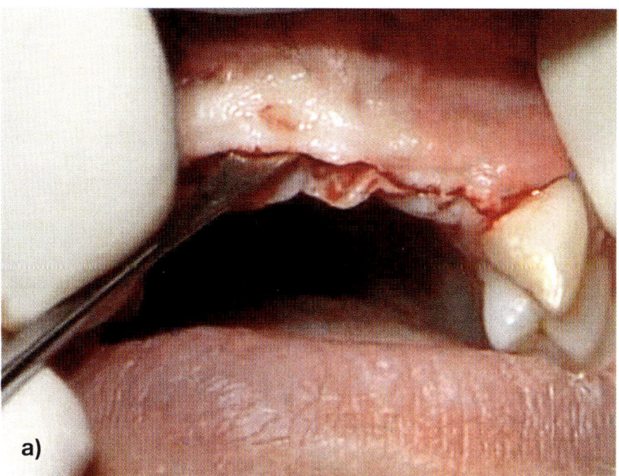

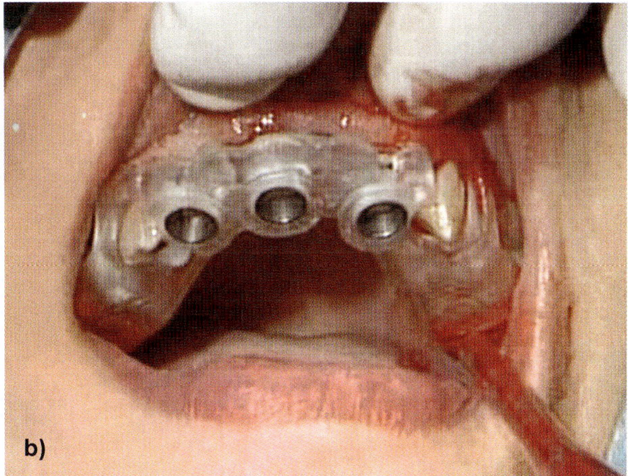

Fig 5-57 (a and b) A full-thickness flap is slightly reflected and elevated, avoiding the releasing of incisions. The surgical guide is then placed and stabilized.

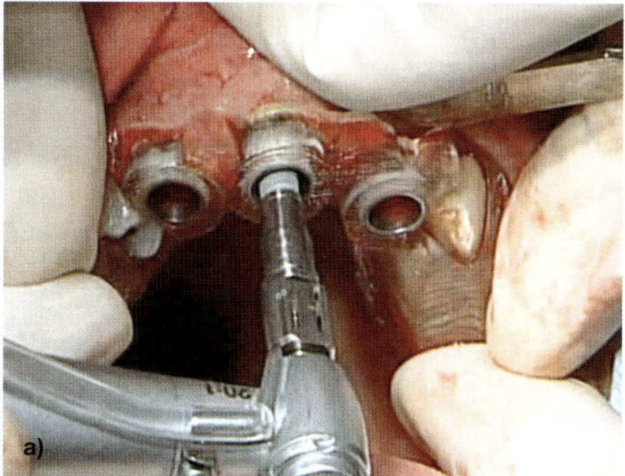

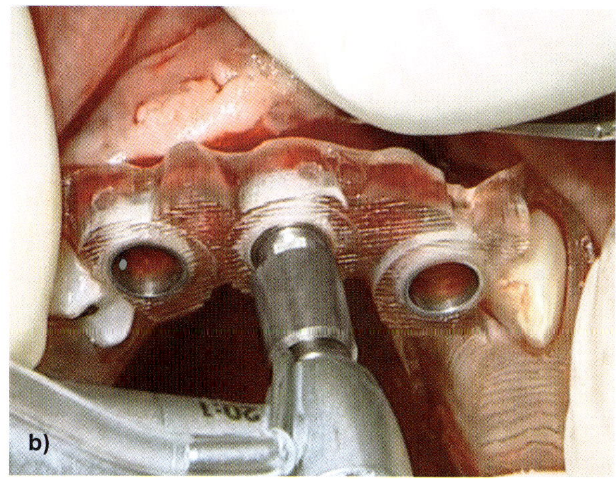

Fig 5-58 (a and b) Drilling sequences and implant placement. The hand piece should be firmly handled to avoid any slight angulation when inserting the implants.

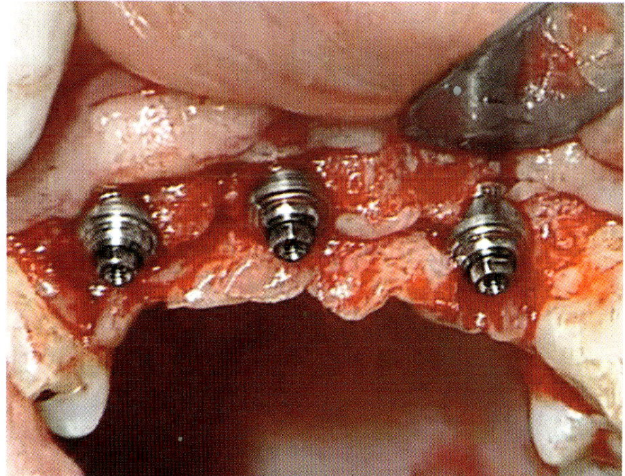

Fig 5-59 The implants are placed; three multi-unit abutments are inserted.

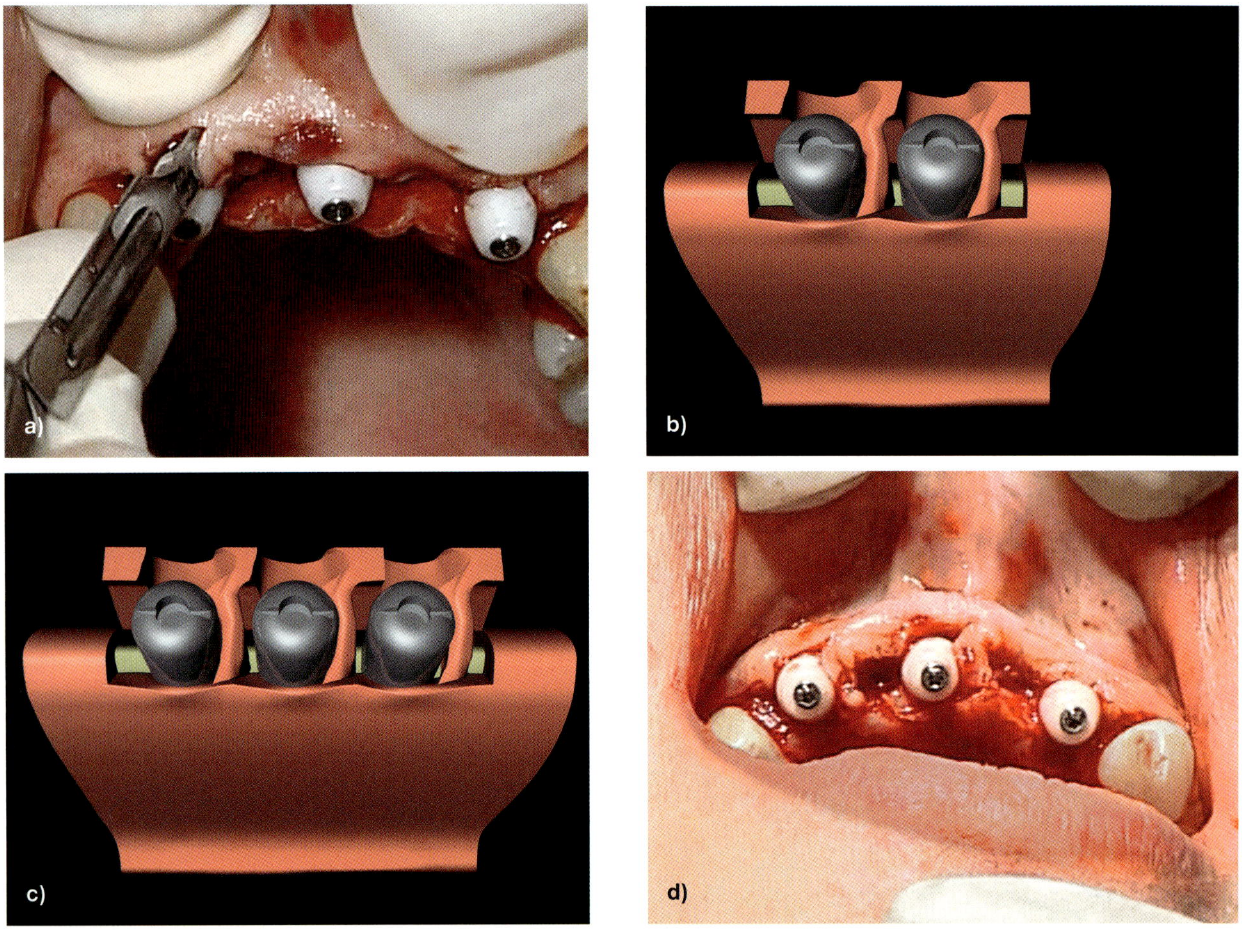

Fig 5-60 (a–d) The papillæ regeneration technique is applied to recreate a more favorable peri-implant soft tissue environment.

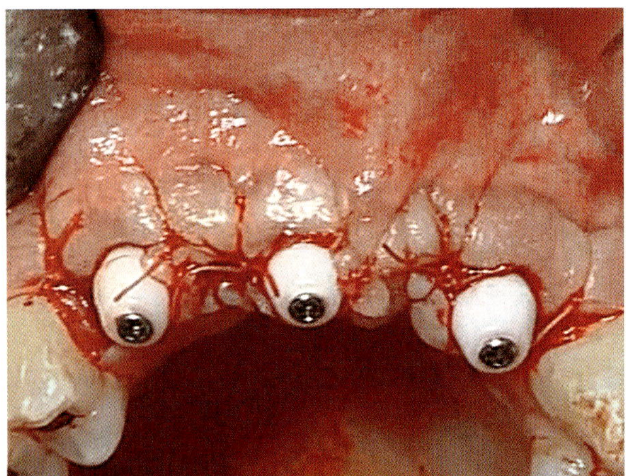

Fig 5-61 Mattress sutures above the papillæ are used to stabilize the tissues into position.

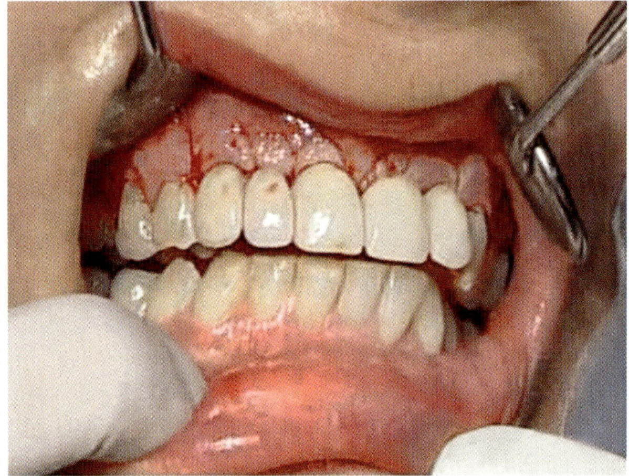

Fig 5-62 With the fixed partial denture in place, note the optimal tissue adaptation to the prosthetic restoration.

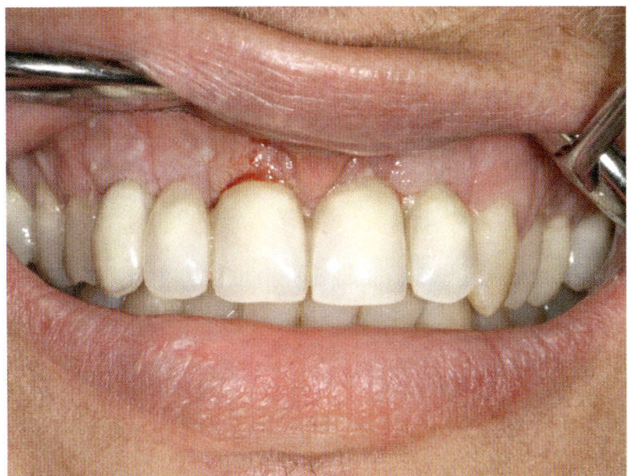

Fig 5-63 Healing after 4 weeks.

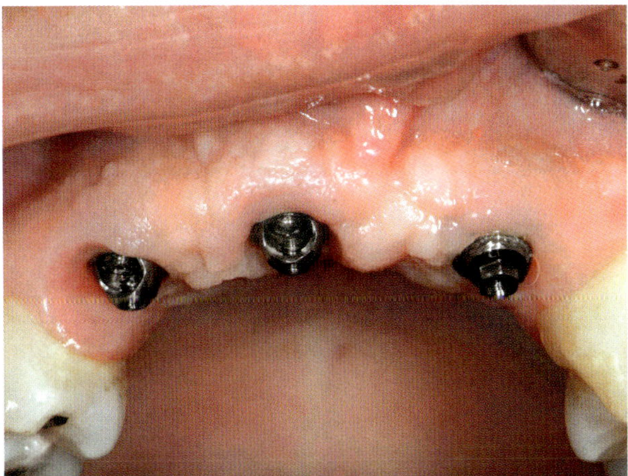

Fig 5-64 Four months later, the fixed partial denture is removed. Note the aspect of the soft tissue surrounding the abutments; 17-degree abutments have been placed to give more space for the cosmetic material when constructing the anterior fixed partial denture.

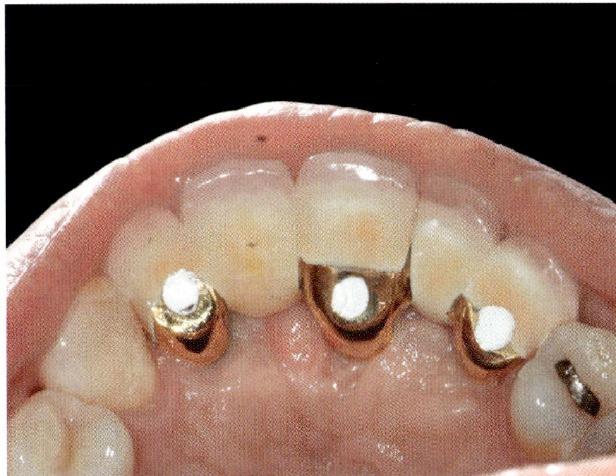

Fig 5-65 Occlusal view. Note the support and translucency of the porcelain, and optimal position of the implants.

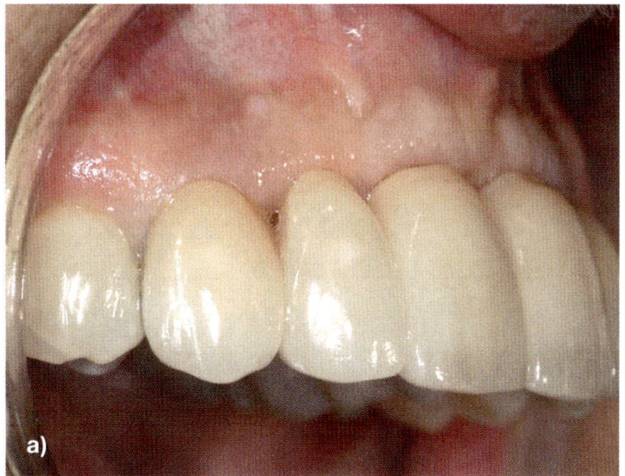

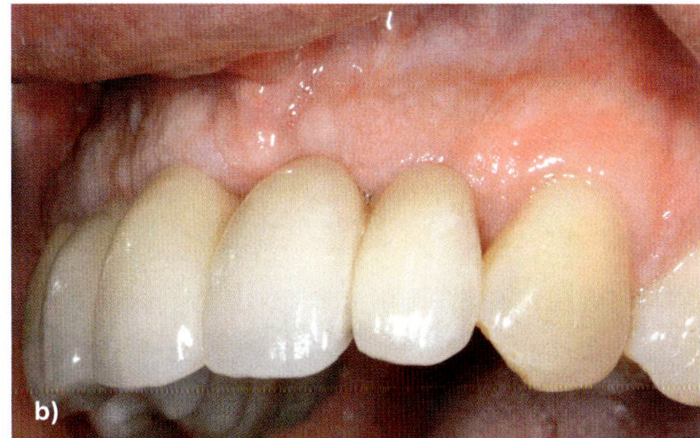

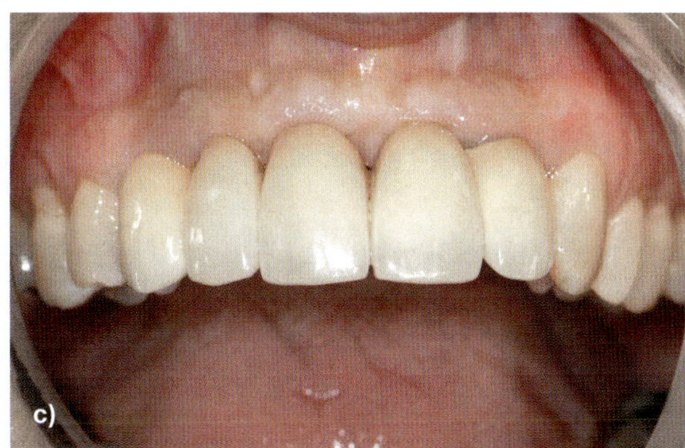

Fig 5-66 (a–c) Lateral and anterior views of the implant-supported fixed partial denture.

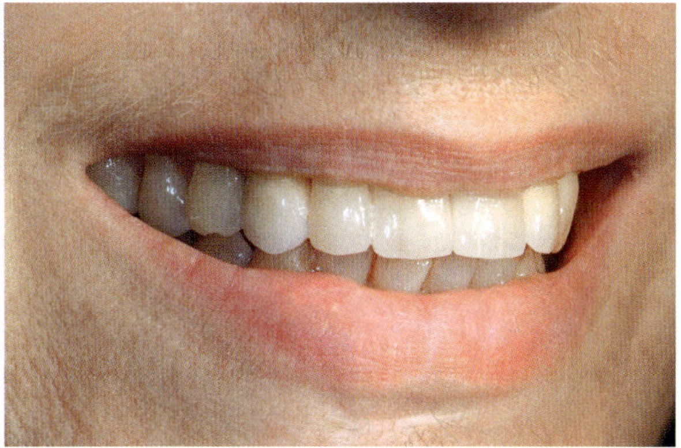

Fig 5-67 Clinical situation 1 year after implant surgery.

Further reading

Adell R, Lekholm U, Brånemark P-I. Surgical procedures. In: Brånemark PI, Zarb GA, Albrektsson T (eds). Tissue-integrated prostheses: osseointegration in clinical dentistry. Chicago: Quintessence, 1985:211-232.

Andreasen JO, Kristerson L, Nilson H, Dahlin K, Schwartz O, Palacci P et al. Implants in the anterior region. In: Andreasen JO, Andreasen FM (eds). Textbook and color atlas of traumatic injuries to the teeth, 3rd edition. Copenhagen: Munksgaard, 1993.

Bengazi F, Wennström JL, Lekholm U. Recession of the soft tissue margin at oral implants. A 2-year longitudinal prospective study. Clin Oral Implants Res 1996;7:303-310.

Berglundh T, Lindhe J. Dimension of the peri-implant mucosa. Biological width revisited. J Clin Periodontol 1996;23:971-973.

Hertel RC, Blijdorp PA, Kalk W, Baker DL. Stage 2 surgical techniques in endosseous implantation. Int J Oral Maxillofac Implants 1994;9:273-278.

Israelsson H, Plemons JM. Dental implants, regenerative techniques, and periodontal plastic surgery to restore maxillary anterior esthetics. Int J Oral Maxillofac Implants 1993;8:555-561.

Kenney EB, Weinlander M, Moy PK. Uncovering implant. A review of the UCLA modification of second stage surgical technique for uncovering implants. J Calif Dent Assoc 1989;3:18-22.

Liljenberg B, Gualini F, Berglundh T, Tonetti T, Lindhe J. Some characteristics of the ridge mucosa before and after implant installation. A prospective study in humans. J Clin Periodontol 1996;23:1008-1013.

Moy PK, Weinlænder M, Kenney EB. Soft tissue modifications of surgical techniques for placement and uncovering of osseointegrated implants. Dent Clin North Am 1989; 33:665-681.

Palacci P. Amenagement des tissus peri-implantaires intéret de la regeneration des papilles. Real Clin 1992;3:381-387.

Palacci P. Optimal implant positioning and soft tissue management for the Brånemark system. Chicago: Quintessence, 1995.

Palacci P. Optimal implant positioning and soft-tissue considerations. Oral Maxillofac Surg Clin North Am 1996; 8:445-452.

Palacci P, Ericsson I. Esthetic implant dentistry. Chicago: Quintessence, 2001.

Seibert J, Lindhe J. Esthetics in Periodontal Therapy. In: Lindhe J, Karring T, Lang NP (eds). Clinical periodontology and implant dentistry, 3rd edition. Copenhagen: Munksgaard, 1997:647-681.

Strub JP, Garberthuel TW, Grunder U. The role of attached gingiva in the health of peri-implant tissues in dogs. Int J Periodontics Restorative Dent 1991;11:317-333.

Sullivan D, Kay H, Schwartz M, Gelb D. Esthetic problems in the anterior maxilla. Int J Oral Maxillofac Implants 1994; 9(Suppl):64-74.

Wennström JL, Bengazi F, Lekholm U. The influence of the masticatory mucosa on the peri-implant soft tissue condition. Clin Oral Implants Res 1994;5:1-8.

Chapter 6

NobelGuide prostheses

Pelle Pettersson, Christer Dagnelid

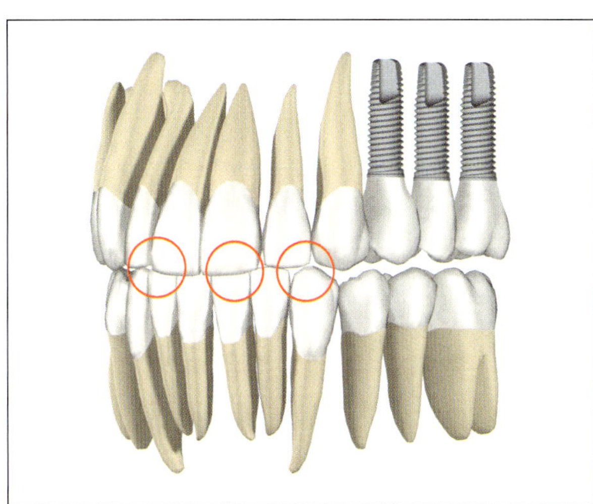

The final treatment outcome of NobelGuide is an absolute reflection of the radiographic guide. Therefore, accurate design of the radiographic guide is a prerequisite for a successful treatment. This chapter outlines the prosthetic parameters that constitute the basis for the radiographic guide, the surgical guide and, thereby, the end result of the NobelGuide treatment. Attention is given to the edentulous maxilla reconstruction planned using radiographic computerized tomography (CT).

General factors for quality assurance

As for every implant-supported restoration special care must be taken with:

- case documentation: medical and dental history, complete oral and dental examination, study casts, photographic records, radiographic examinations
- choice of method and products
- communication: with the patient and dental team, within the dental team
- use of evidence-based practice
- medico-legal aspects
- signed informed consent.

Preparations

To optimize the treatment outcome, it is crucial to establish a proper level of oral hygiene, and to be sure that possible periodontal lesions within the opposing dentition are adequately treated.

Extraction of the remaining roots must be done with great care in a non-traumatic way so that the buccal bone walls of the alveolars are preserved. This often involves the use of a periotome. Traumatized or destroyed labial bone walls may negatively affect the final positioning of the implants and the overall treatment outcome.

In the worst-case scenario, severely impaired buccal bone walls may compromise the use of NobelGuide.

To obtain the correct radiographic information covering hard and soft tissue during the planned CT procedure, it is important to allow adequate bone healing. The length of this healing period is different for each patient, taking from weeks to several months depending on the soft and hard tissue conditions of each individual. As CT exposes the patient to significant irradiation, it is recommended to take intraoral radiographs to verify bone healing before performing CT.

During CT, the radiographic guide is used to simulate the teeth, the architecture/outline of the gingival tissue, the mucosa and the edentulous spaces. The radiographic guide may be based on an already existing denture, but it is preferable to base this on the immediate denture used during postextraction healing.

The radiographic guide

NobelGuide computer-based planning can be used for single tooth loss or for the treatment of partially and fully edentulous patients. It is crucial to have a sufficient amount of bone and be sure that the bone has fully recovered after extractions or hard/ soft tissue grafting procedures. The patient's ability to open the mouth to accommodate the surgical procedure must be checked before surgery.

Once the initial preparation, extractions and periodontal treatment have occurred, and sufficient healing time has passed, the radiographic guide can be prepared. For a fully edentulous patient the existing denture can be optimized. However, if this is not possible, a new one needs to be fabricated. In single tooth loss and partially edentulous patients, the laboratory will fabricate an acrylic radiographic guide.

The clinician should take an alginate impression of the opposing jaw and take two bite registration indexes in a stiff silicone material. One index should be used to support the jaws in the correct occlusion during CT; the other index should be sent to the dental laboratory to be used when fabricating the final implant-supported fixed partial denture.

The bite registration must be horizontally well balanced. If there are only a few teeth remaining in the opposing jaw, the edentulous area is filled with a stiff putty material or a temporary partial denture is made for support. The radiographic guide should be fabricated in acrylic.

General design requirements of the radiographic guide

The radiographic guide should:

- show an optimal representation of position of teeth to be restored
- be an optimal fit to anatomy including palate (if applicable), gingiva/mucosa and existing denture (if applicable), and covering buccal, lingual and occclusal aspects
- extend over the buccal and lingual soft tissue to the full depth of the vestibular area in edentulous areas
- have an ideal set up of teeth in terms of occlusion, position, occlusal height and lip support
- include inspection windows for partial and single edentulous situations
- be made in a non-radiopaque material, i.e. acrylic
- extend back to the retro-molar area for good support
- include between six and nine gutta-percha markers.

Designing the radiographic guide

Clinicians should consider the functional, geometrical and mechanical requirements of the surgical template when designing the radiographic guide. In fully edentulous patients, the existing optimized prosthesis or a specially produced prosthesis where the teeth are optimally placed for esthetics, phonetics and vertical height could be used.

A sufficient part of the soft tissue should be covered to allow for placement of the guided anchor pin. The anchor pin should have a large enough base of thick material for optimal stiffness of the anchor pin sleeve. This can be verified using Procera software.

In single and partially edentulous patients, stone models based on the alginate impressions will need to be fabricated. The stone models will need to be set up in the articulator using the bite registration index.

A diagnostic wax-up should be made of the patient's tooth/teeth to be restored on the stone model. Existing teeth are covered down to the vestibular extension with a 2.5–3 mm thick resin material (acrylic). If applicable, the palate should also be covered. The clinician must be sure to block all undercuts. Buccal, lingual and occlusal sides should be covered for optimal retention, as this is transferred to the surgical template. The clinician should leave the occlusal aspects of areas to be restored untouched, and cover only the buccal and lingual aspects with acrylic material. This is a required so that the correct occlusal plane is transferred to the Procera software.

Preparing and fabricating the radiographic guide (for all indications)

The clinician should undertake the following steps:

- attach the resin to cover the lingual and buccal sides of the diagnostic wax-up without adding material on the occlusal aspect of the wax-up
- ensure an optimal and homogenous bond between wax-up and acrylic
- ensure that the radiographic guide extends all the way back to rest on the retro-molar area
- consider the following option: the set-up of teeth can also be made of acrylic as long as the geometry is optimal
- make the radiographic guide of homogenous and uniform acrylic, which is beneficial during CT.

Reference points (for all indications)

To facilitate the double CT technique and the subsequent matching of the two CT scans in the Procera software, between six and nine reference points must be inserted into the radiographic guide.

- Six small holes, 1 mm deep and 1.5 mm in diameter, are made in the radiographic guide.
- Two of the reference points are placed lingually/palatally to the canines, two distally/buccally to the premolars and two in the molar region.
- The reference points are placed at different levels in relation to the occlusal plane.
- The holes are filled with gutta-percha.
- In single and partially edentulous patients where metal fillings are present in the existing dentition, the reference points are placed on levels other than those of the fillings, e.g. apically to or between the roots.

Inspection windows (partially and single edentulous patients)

The following steps should be undertaken.

- Inspection windows made on single and partial radiographic guides are transferred to the surgical template. This allows inspection of the underlying dentition, thus confirming proper seating of the surgical template during fixture installation.
- Inspection windows are made in the radiographic guide through the occlusal surface over the existing dentition.
- Three or four windows are created, evenly distributed over the entire arch, with one or two windows located adjacent to the area to be restored.
- The inspection windows should preferably be placed over a cusp or a corner of a tooth so that the underlying dentition protrudes through the window.

Radiographic index

For fully edentulous patients, the bite registration in stiff silicone is the radiographic index to be used during CT. In partially and single edentulous patients, the radiographic index is prepared by inserting the radiographic guide in the articulator; using stiff putty material, the clinician makes an occlusal index between the radiographic guide and the opposing dentition. If the patient only has a few teeth in the opposing jaw and does not wear a partial denture, the clinician should be sure to fill up the area where the teeth are missing with stiff putty material to make contact with the alveolar ridge. This is to ensure that there is a horizontal, well-balanced bite registration. An alternative is to fabricate a provisional partial denture replacing the missing teeth and thus facilitate an optimal bite-registration.

Once the radiographic index has been established (for all indications), the patient can be referred for CT. A referring form can be written out from the Procera software, where the patient has been registered and given a unique identification code. The radiographic guide and the radiographic index are delivered to the radiographer to be placed intraorally during the CT examination.

The CT scan, Procera software for planning and 'computer surgery' and the surgical protocol have been discussed in Chapters 2 to 4.

NobelGuide prosthetic solutions

1. If one tooth is missing, a temporary restoration will be delivered at implant placement. After proper healing of soft and hard tissue, a Procera crown with an individual abutment will be placed for proper esthetics.
2. With multiple missing teeth, a temporary solution is also preferred (screw-retained or temporarily cemented to abutments).
3. For fully edentulous patients, the final fixed prosthesis – a Procera Implant Bridge (i.e. a milled titanium framework dressed with acrylic "gums" and teeth) – will be placed directly following implant placement. Alternatively, a full acrylic temporary bridge can be placed at the time of surgery, to be followed later by a Procera Implant Bridge with individualized high-esthetic porcelain.

As occlusion is critical for success when applying immediate loading, special care should be taken with this aspect of the treatment. The occlusal design of the implant-supported fixed restoration

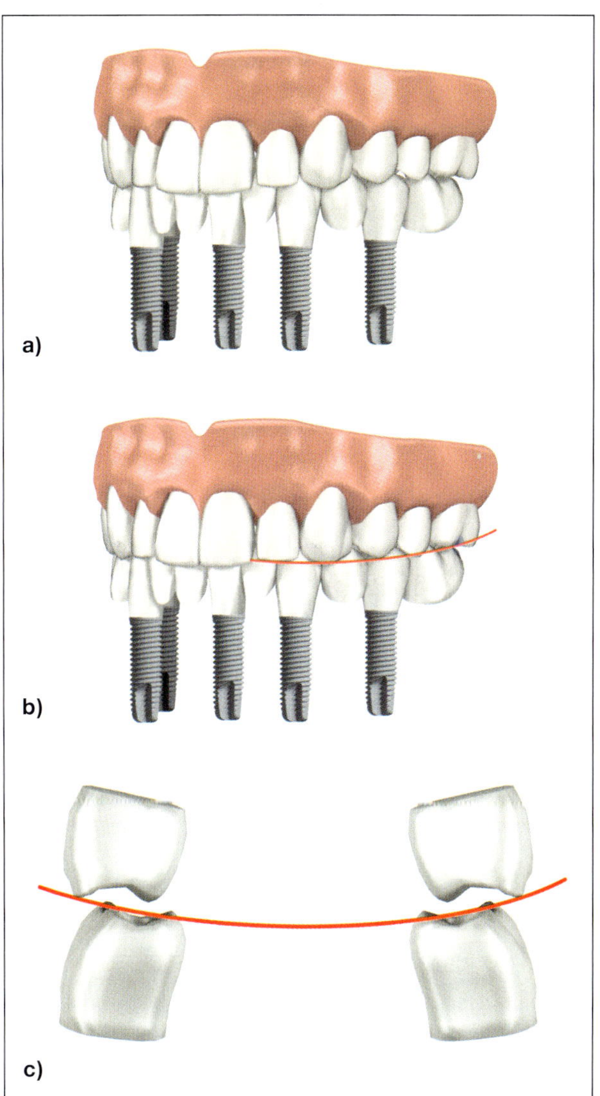

Fig 6-1 (a–c) The opposite jaw is a full removable denture. It is, therefore, desirable that the inter-occlusal relationship is based on a fully balanced occlusion to stabilize the opposing denture.

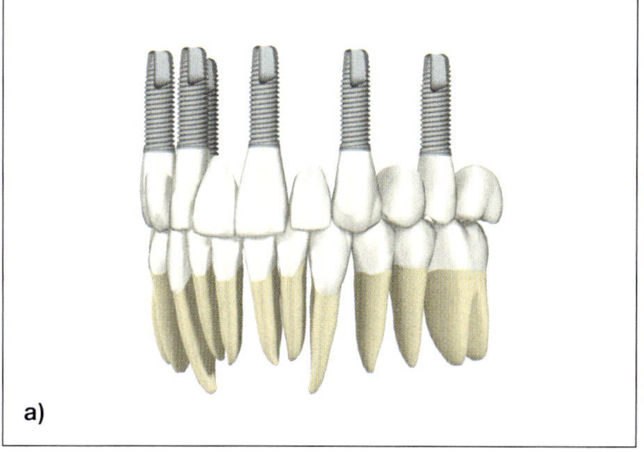

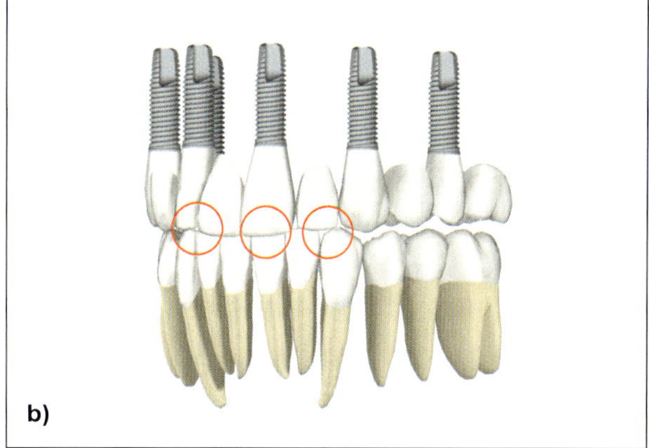

Fig 6-2 (a and b) The opposing dentition is a fixed full bridge/full natural dentition. The preferred approach is, therefore, a group function/anterior guidance situation using flat cusps and with a minimum of extension cantilevers.

should be as close to optimal occlusal relationships as possible, taking into account the features and limitations of the NobelGuide concept. Generally, attention should be paid to the Spee and Wilson curves as well as the Monson plane.

Another general rule is that, irrespective of what type of dentition is present in the opposing jaw, contact on a sole tooth has to be avoided. This means that, for example, a canine rise situation on a NobelGuide fixed partial denture should be avoided.

A third rule is always to use flat cusps on an implant-supported fixed partial denture.

Below are a few examples of occlusal schemes related to various types of tooth loss.

Example 1. If the opposite jaw has a full removable denture, it is desirable that the inter-occlusal

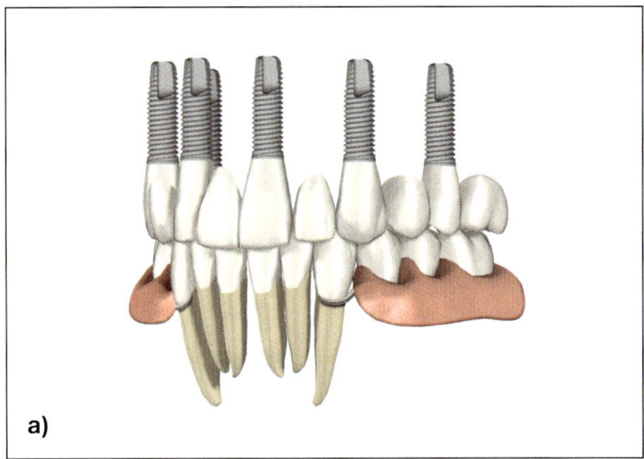

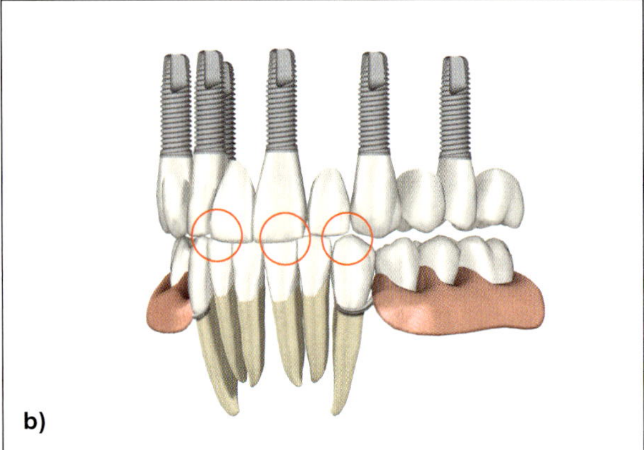

Fig 6-3 (a and b) The opposing dentition is fixed teeth with a removable partial denture: in this case, natural canines and incisors in the lower arch in combination with a mandibular posterior removable partial denture facing a maxillary NobelGuide fixed full arch prosthesis.

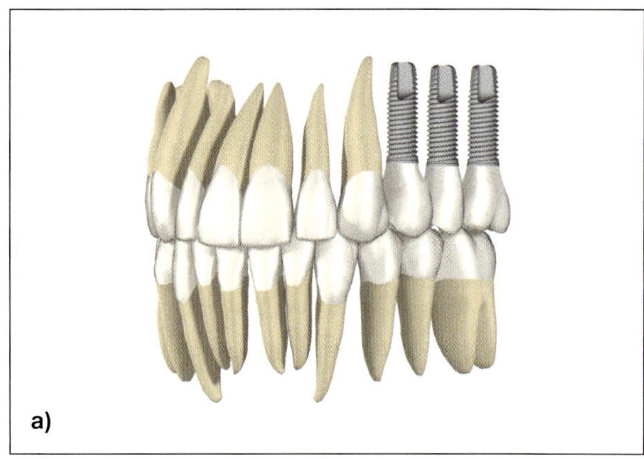

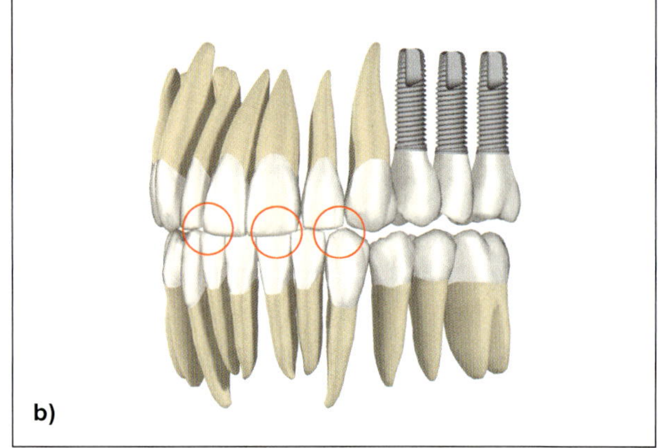

Fig 6-4 (a and b) An implant-supported fixed partial denture based on NobelGuide, opposing a fixed natural dentition: the implant-supported fixed partial denture should make contact only in centric.

relationship is based on a fully balanced occlusion to stabilize the opposing denture (Fig 6-1). To achieve a fully balanced occlusion, it is imperative that the Spee and Wilson curves are respected.

Example 2. If the opposing dentition is a fixed full bridge/full natural dentition (Fig 6-2), the preferred approach is a group function/anterior guidance situation using flat cusps and with a minimum of extension cantilevers.

Example 3. If the opposing dentition has fixed teeth and a removable partial denture (e.g. natural canines and incisors in the lower arch in combination with a mandibular posterior removable partial denture facing a maxillary NobelGuide fixed full arch prosthesis; Fig 6-3), the anterior mandibular natural teeth are used to create a situation of anterior guidance towards the implant-supported fixed full bridge in the maxilla.

Example 4. If an implant-supported fixed partial denture based on NobelGuide is opposing a fixed natural dentition (Fig 6-4), the implant-supported fixed partial denture should make contact only in centric. In laterotrusion/protrusion the implant-supported fixed partial denture should be fully discluded.

Postoperative care and follow-up

Immediately after insertion of the crown or fixed partial denture, intraoral radiographs should be taken for every implant site to confirm that the fit between implant and abutment is perfect. If the fit is not perfect, some peri-implant mucosa may have been trapped during seating of the fixed partial denture. In such cases, the construction has to be removed and corrections made with a tissue punch or scalpel. New radiographs should be taken. When the insertion is screw retained, the abutment screws should be inserted with 35 Ncm torque. Temporary fillings will then be put in the screw holes.

A rough calibration of the occlusion will be made directly after insertion. As the patient is under local anesthesia, a more thorough adjustment will be performed 1 or 2 days after surgery. The goal is a bilaterally well-balanced occlusion with flat cusps, thus avoiding overloading of individual implants.

In the first week, the patient will rinse with chlorhexidine solution. After that, intraoral hygiene information and instruction should be introduced. An electric toothbrush, dental floss and inter-dental brushes are recommended.

Check-ups should be conducted at 1 week, 2 months, 3 months, 6 months and yearly, depending on co-operation from the patient. If there is any sign of bruxism, it is crucial to fabricate a soft or hard night-guard to allow proper osseointegration of the implants.

After 4 weeks, the temporary fillings should be removed. Final tightening of the abutment screws with 35 Ncm torque will be done. Occlusion should be checked at each follow-up visit. The fixed prosthesis should not be removed before 3 months. If a second restoration is needed, the clinician should wait at least 4 months after the initial surgery. The temporary fixed partial denture will be used as a guide for occlusion, function, speech and esthetics.

Case presentations: a prosthetic approach

Case I: edentulous maxilla

A 60-year-old male, in good health and general condition, was referred from his general practitioner for implant treatment in the maxilla. An old porcelain-fused-to-metal (PFM) fixed partial denture had failed through caries and periodontal problems. His mandible was treated with a cross-arch PFM fixed partial denture by the referring dentist. The treatment plan for the maxilla was extractions followed by immediate denture and implant treatment according to the Teeth-in-an-Hour concept. The patient was a famous actor who demanded an immediate solution with fixed teeth (Figs 6-5 and 6-6).

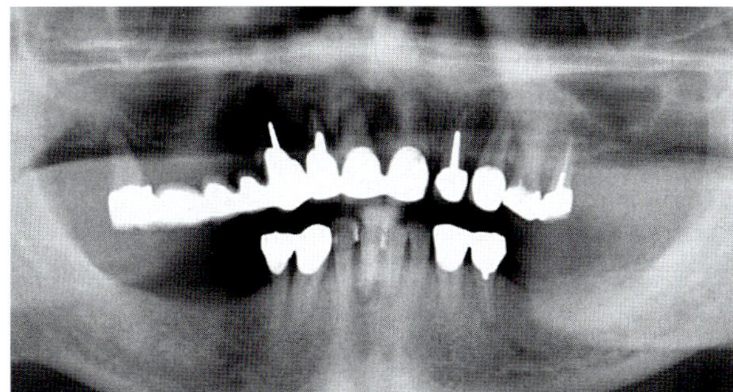

Fig 6-5 Preoperative orthopantomogram showing failed maxillary porcelain-fused-to-metal (PFM) fixed partial denture as a result of caries and periodontal disease. The mandible is seen before treatment with a cross-arch fixed PFM fixed partial denture.

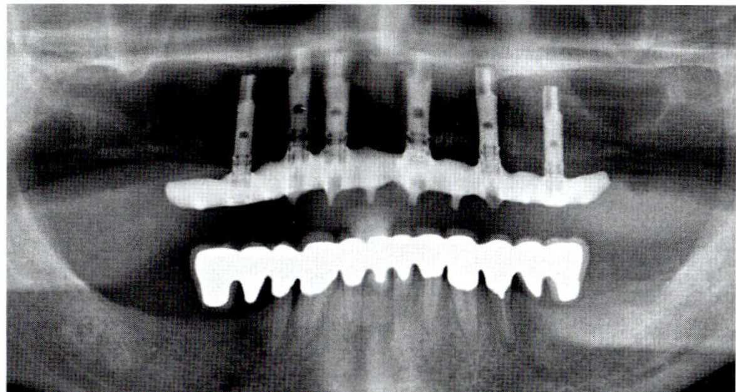

Fig 6-6 Orthopantomogram taken after surgical and prosthetic treatment in both jaws.

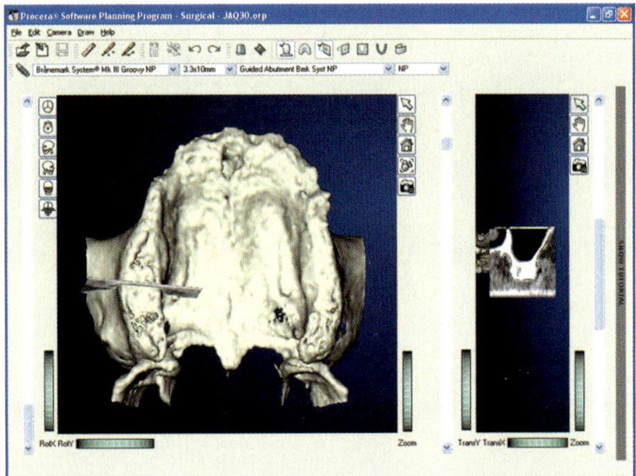

Fig 6-7 Three-dimensional model of patient's bone, recreated using Procera software from axial re-slices taken by computerized tomography. Bone anatomy shows adequate properties to apply the immediate loading protocol using the Teeth-in-an-Hour concept.

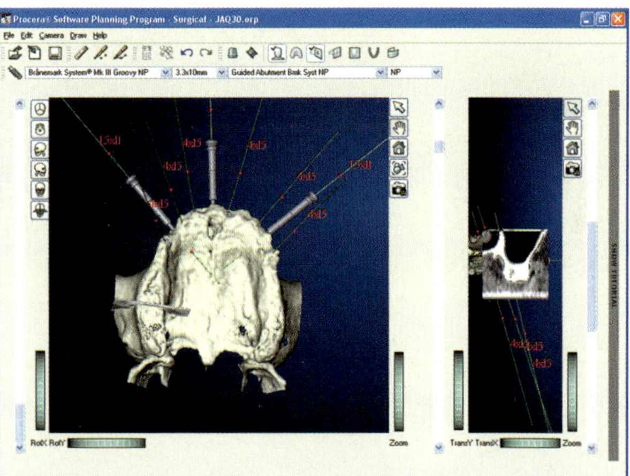

Fig 6-8 Finished surgical planning seen in Procera software. The six Brånemark Mk III 4.0 mm implants are evenly distributed along the alveolar arch.

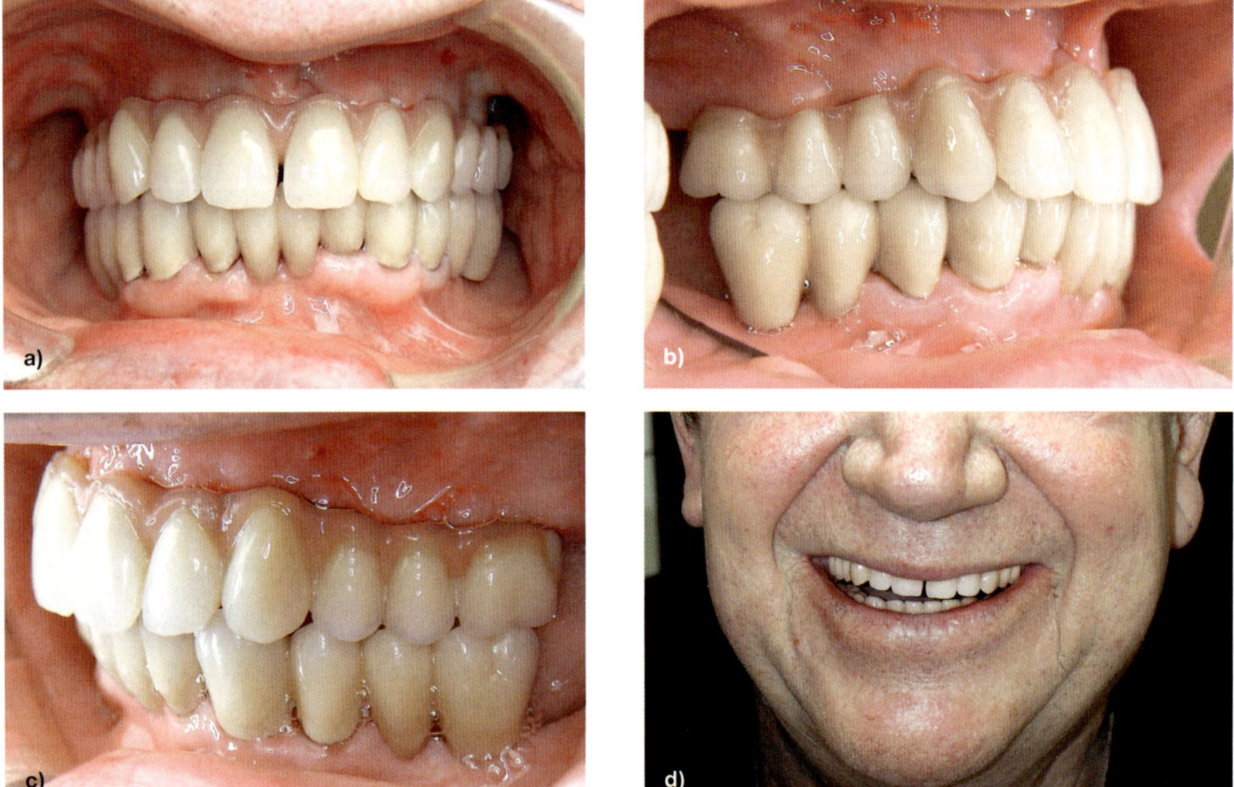

Fig 6-9 (a–d) Postoperative photographs. An individualized tooth set-up has been used according to the patient's request. The diastema between the central incisors reproduces the original dentition set-up. Lateral views show a balanced occlusion, designed and kept from the previous radiographic guide and copied by the dental technician. Although speech difficulties are seldom a problem, owing to the patient's profession, it was important not to overextend the palatal aspect of the fixed partial denture, thus avoiding any speech problems.

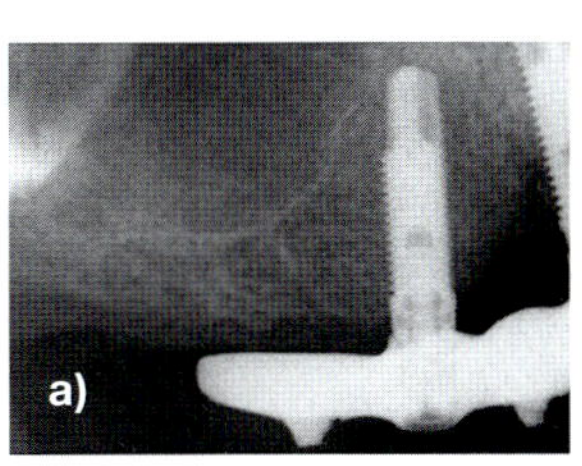

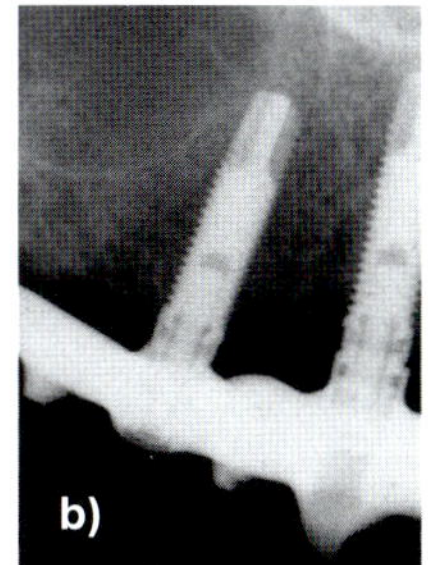

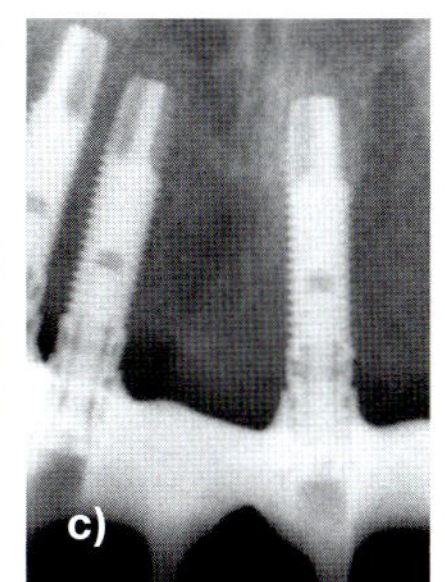

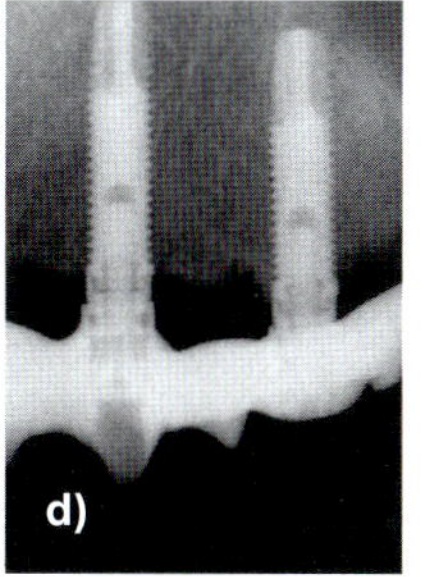

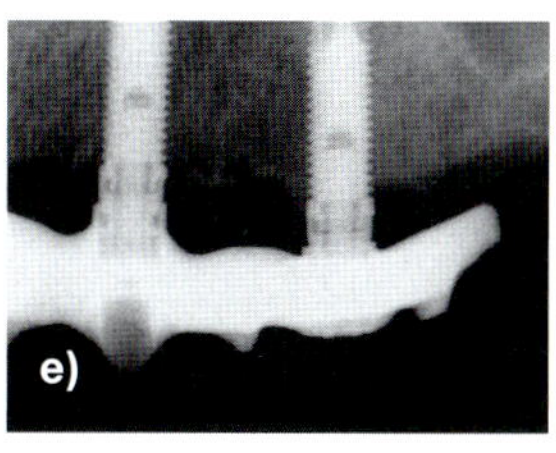

Fig 6-10 (a–e) Intraoral radiographs taken after surgery to verify the proper fit between guided abutments and implants. A comparison can also be made regarding the placement of the implants in the patient's bone. The surgical planning in Procera software compared with the radiographs shows a similar relation to both the sinus and incisor canal.

The initial intraoral examination and radiograph evaluation revealed an acceptable quantity and quality of alveolar bone. Because of the patient's career, prosthetic planning was vital (Figs 6-7 and 6-8). The patient requested an individualized teeth set-up, both keeping the original look and facilitating phonetics. The clinicians tried to reduce the period between the delivery of the immediate denture and the final Teeth-in-an-Hour to 4 months after extractions. Next, a final hard relining was made and insertion of gutta-percha reference points performed.

After the CT procedure was completed, the results were analyzed using Procera software (Fig 6-7). The alveolar crest showed good height and width, which simplified surgical planning. According to the surgical protocol (Ericsson et al 2000, Ericsson and Nilner 2002), the treatment was planned for six Brånemark Mk III (4.0 mm diameter) implants with the TiUnite surface (Fig 6-8). The implant positions were optimally guided by the prosthetic reconstruction represented by the radiographic guide (in this case, equal to the removable complete denture) and the posterior implants were placed as distal as possible regarding the posterior areas.

The NobelGuide concept allows more superficial placements of the fixtures, which are positioned as parallel as possible, simplifying the connection of the fixed partial denture to the implants immediately following surgery. The angulation restriction between the implants is maximum 30 degrees. The length of the fixtures is guided by the surrounding anatomy. They should be as long as possible without interfering with anatomical structures, such as the nasal cavity or incisor canal.

The final prosthesis for this patient was a Teeth-in-an-Hour reconstruction, made of a Procera Implant Bridge framework and acrylic teeth, designed exactly as the optimized radiographic guide for tooth set-up, color and occlusal design (Fig 6-9).

Intraoral radiographs were taken to verify the proper fit of the abutments to the fixtures (Fig 6-10).

Case II: edentulous maxilla

An 87-year-old male, in good health and general condition, was referred from a general practitioner for an overdenture treatment initially. He had been edentulous in the maxilla and mandible for 15 years. Owing to the biological resorption and loss of denture retention, the patient's wish was for a fixed restoration rather than an overdenture. The mandible was planned according to the Brånemark System (Ericsson et al 2000, Ericsson and Nilner 2002), owing to the severe resorption and the difficulty of using a NobelGuide treatment in these patients (see surgical discussion below).

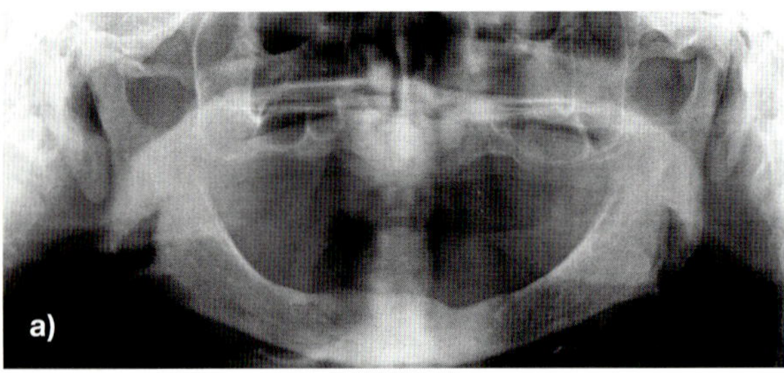

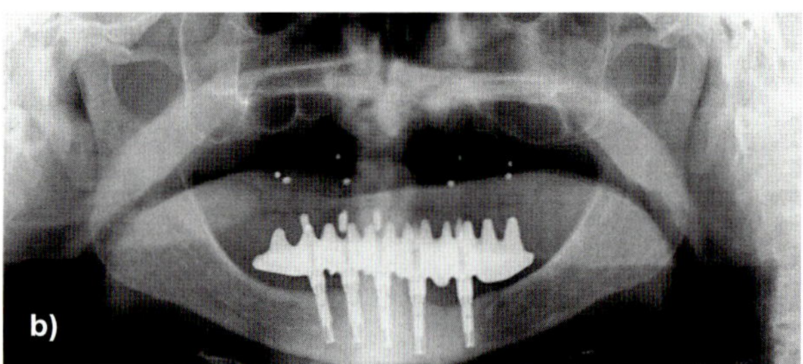

Fig 6-11 (a) Preoperative orthopantomogram (OPG) showing edentulism in both jaws. **(b)** The OPG taken after treatment of the mandible with the Nordic Bridge concept.

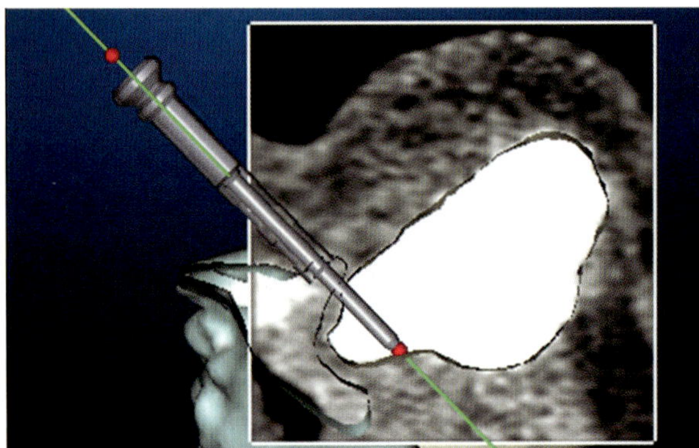

Fig 6-12 Difficulty in placing horizontal anchor pins in the mandible in patients with advanced resorption. This often ends up with an overly vertical placement of the anchor pin.

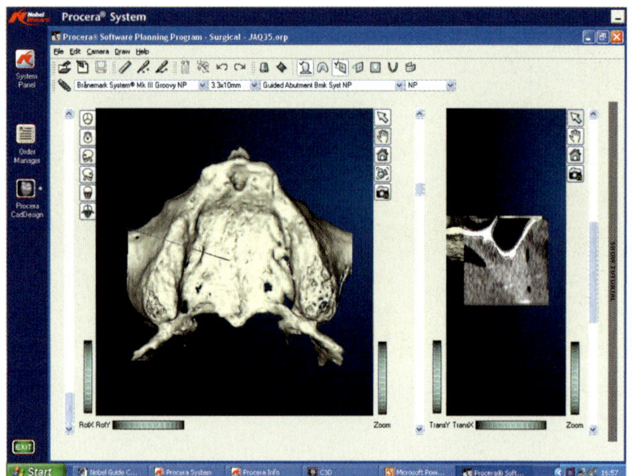

Fig 6-13 Three-dimensional model of the patient's bone, recreated with a Procera software from axial re-slices taken with computerized tomography. Similar to Case I, bone anatomy shows good properties for use of the immediate loading protocol in the Teeth-in-an-Hour concept.

The maxilla was planned for a Teeth-in-an-Hour treatment (Fig 6-11).

Treatment planning involved implant-supported fixed restoration of both jaws. The intention was to start with the mandibular treatment. Owing to the advanced resorption of the alveolar process, the patient experienced severe retention problems with his denture, with very limited vestibular extensions, and a very flat and narrow alveolar crest.

The use of the NobelGuide concept is relatively contraindicated in patients of this type owing to the lack of retention of the surgical template. The anchor pins have to be placed in a more or less vertical direction as the lingual aspect of the mandible should not be penetrated with an anchor pin (Fig 6-12). The prosthetic approach is simplified when establishing the vertical dimension and occlusal plane.

In such patients, the clinician may plan to start with a Nordic Bridge treatment in the mandible. This includes a traditional surgical protocol with placement of five implants between the mental foramina, and the placement of five multi-unit abutments. An impression is taken and the tooth set-up tried in the same day. The supra-construction, a Procera Implant Bridge with acrylic teeth, is delivered within 1 week.

Owing to limited resorption in the maxilla, a NobelGuide treatment according to Teeth-in-an-Hour concept was planned.

The patient's request regarding the tooth set-up was to match his previous fixed partial denture in all

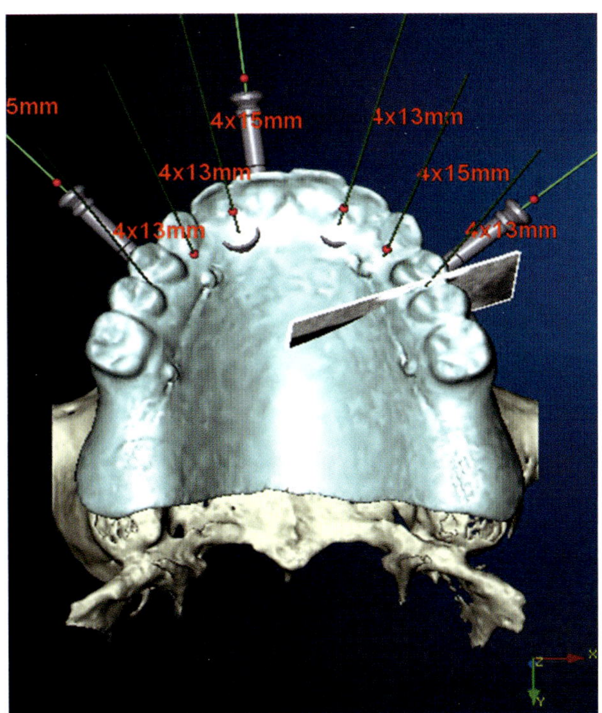

Fig 6-14 Finished surgical planning seen in Procera software. Six Brånemark Mk III 4.0 mm implants have been placed in an even distribution along the alveolar arch.

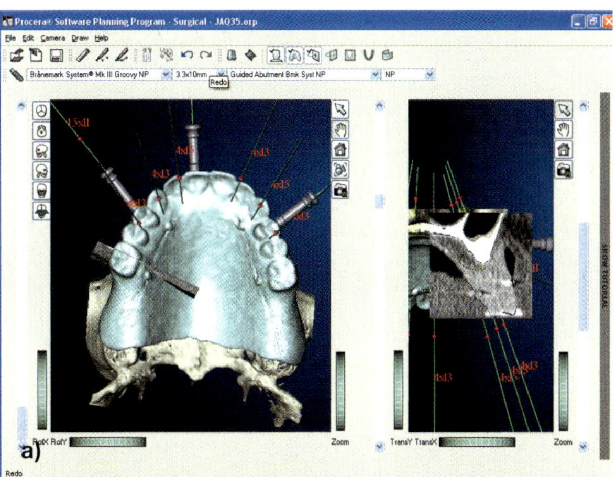

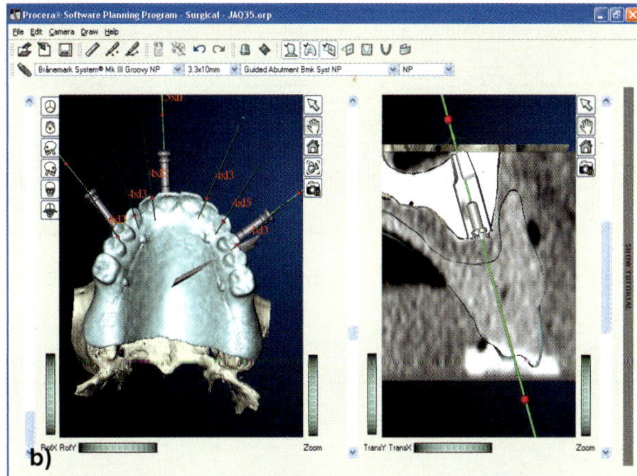

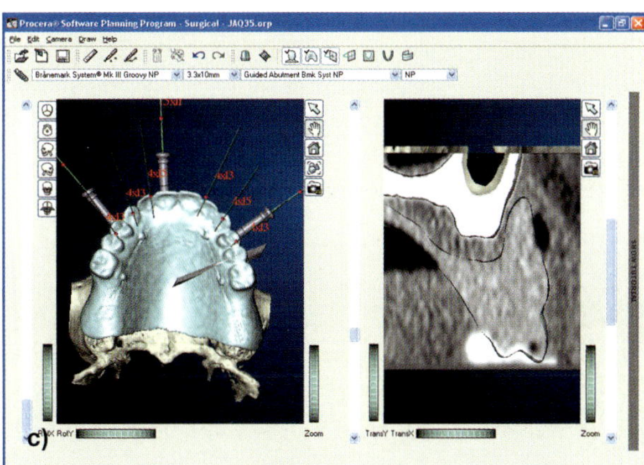

Fig 6-15 (a–c) The most distal implants on both sides had to be placed between the first and second premolar giving unfavorable access holes for screw retention.

aspects. As in many prosthetic treatments, photographs were taken for communication with the dental technician.

It is also important to realize that the design of the radiographic guide determines the final prosthetic outcome.

Procera software analysis revealed a maxilla with a good quantity, quality and height of alveolar bone (Fig 6-13). Again the goal is to place six fixtures in a favorable distribution along the entire arch. If possible, the access holes for the screws are placed in either the middle of the tooth, as in the premolars, or in a palatal position, for the canine and incisor region (Fig 6-14).

In this case, the sinus presented some difficulties, as seen in the planning illustrations (Fig 6-15). Both

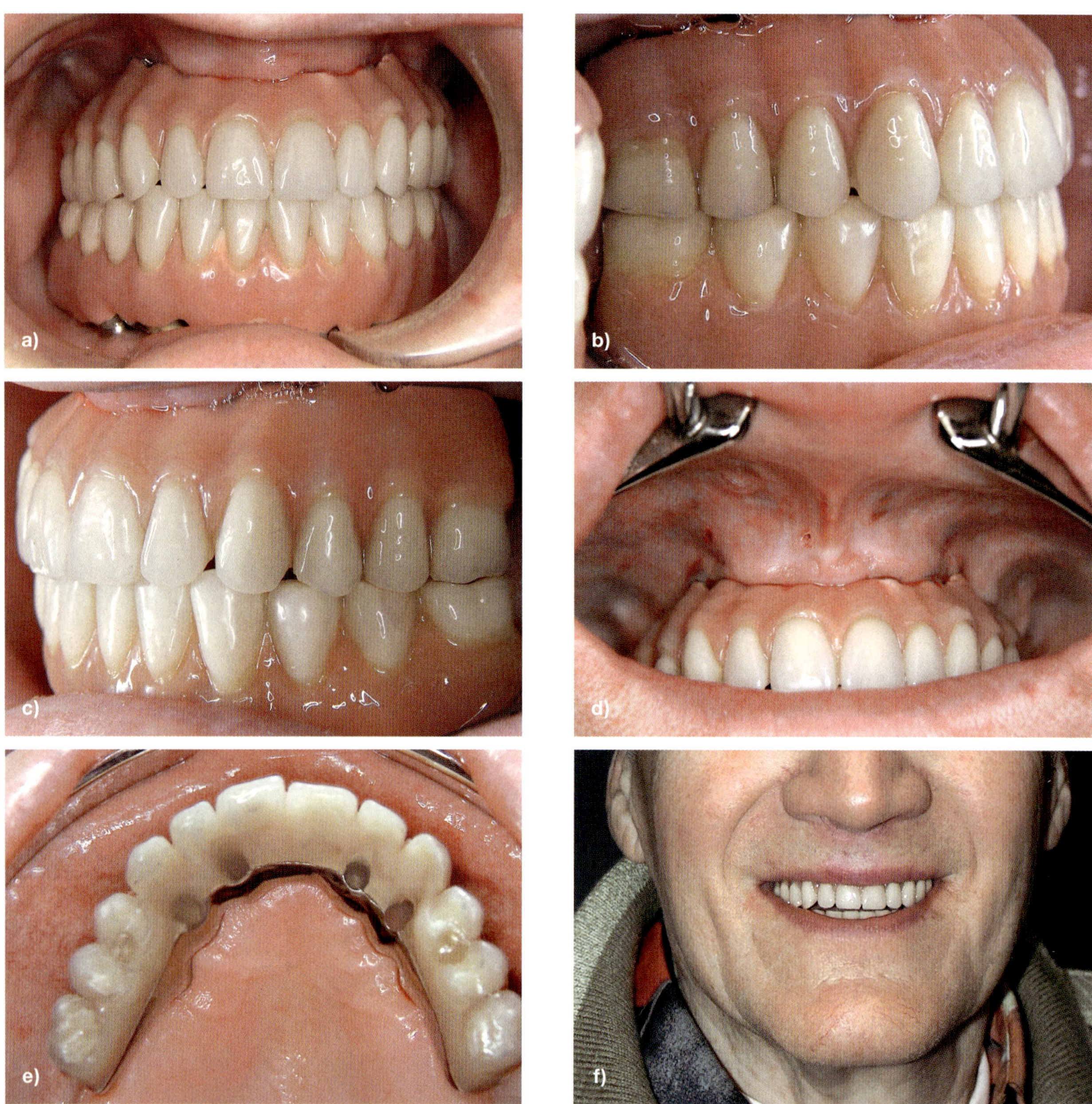

Fig 6-16 (a–f) Postoperative photographs of an individualized tooth set-up according to previous photographs of old fixed partial dentures. Occlusion is designed to be balanced and the fixed partial denture is a Procera Implant Bridge with acrylic teeth. Note that the NobelGuide concept minimizes the surgical trauma. Minimal bleeding may be observed 1 hour after surgery, and the positions of the horizontal anchor pins are the only remaining defects. The occlusal view shows access holes in the most distal implant positions.

the right and left sides of these images show the final position of the access holes between the first and second premolars.

Even though a more angulated position could have given a better outcome, the goal is to minimize the difference in angulation as much as possible to simplify the installation of the fixed partial denture after surgery. More superficial placements than in a traditional protocol can be seen in this case.

As for Case I, the final reconstruction is a Procera Implant Bridge with acrylic teeth. Immediately after surgery, intraoral radiographs were taken to verify the proper fit between implants and abutments (Figs 6-16 and 6-17).

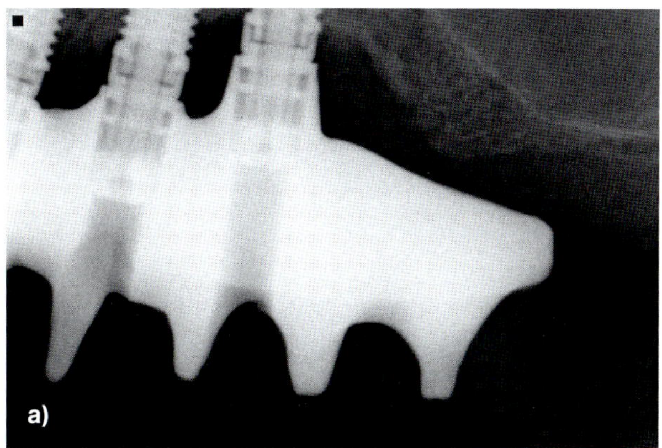

Fig 6-17 (a–f) Intraoral radiographs taken after surgery to verify the proper fit between the guided abutments and implants. Optimal fit is observed at all sites.

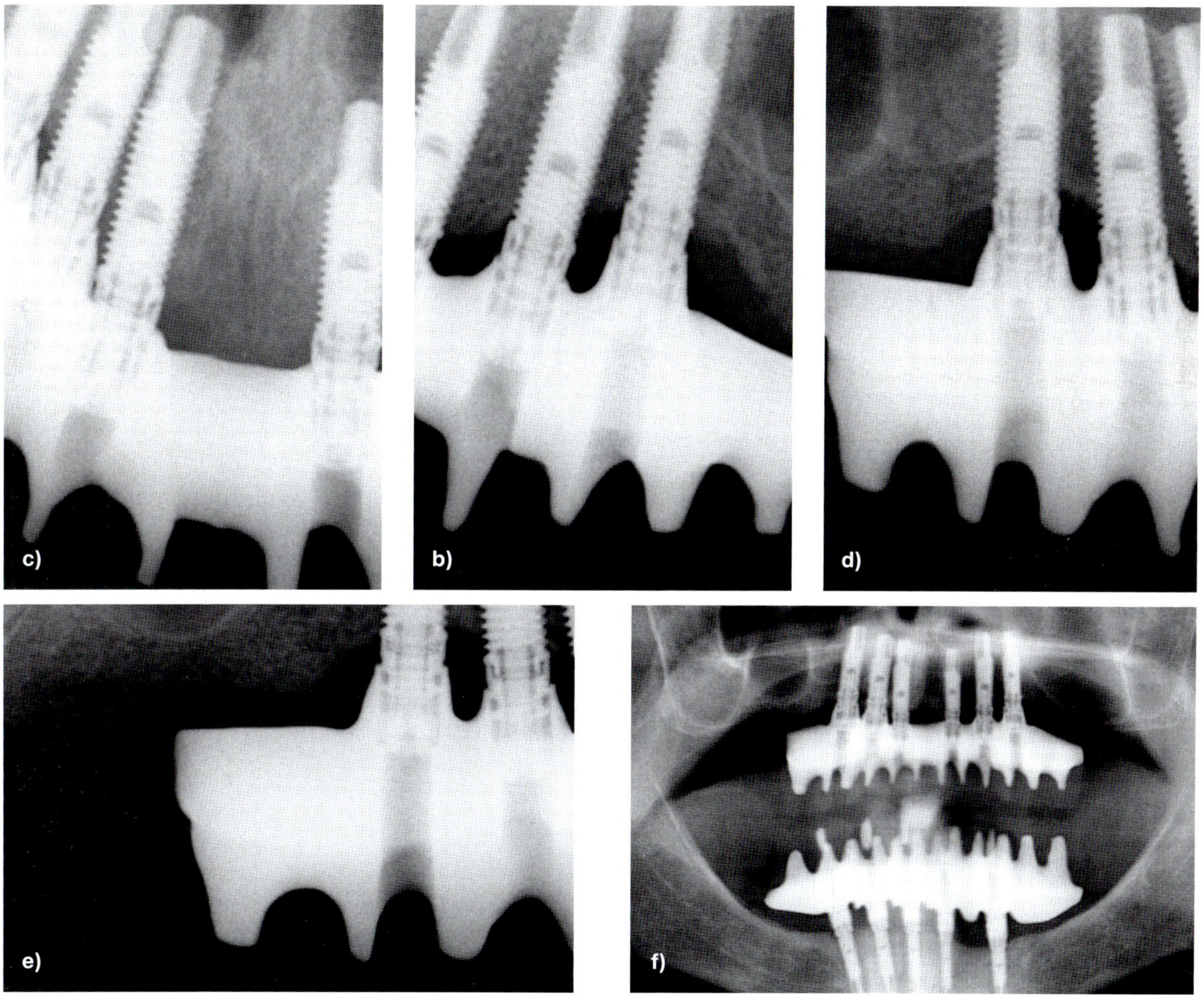

References

Ericsson I, Randow K, Nilner K, Petersson A. Early functional loading of Brånemark dental implants. A 5-year follow-up study. Clin Implant Dent Rel Res 2000;2:70-77.

Ericsson I, Nilner K. Early functional loading using Brånemark dental implants. Int J Periodontics Restorative Dent 2002:22:9-19.

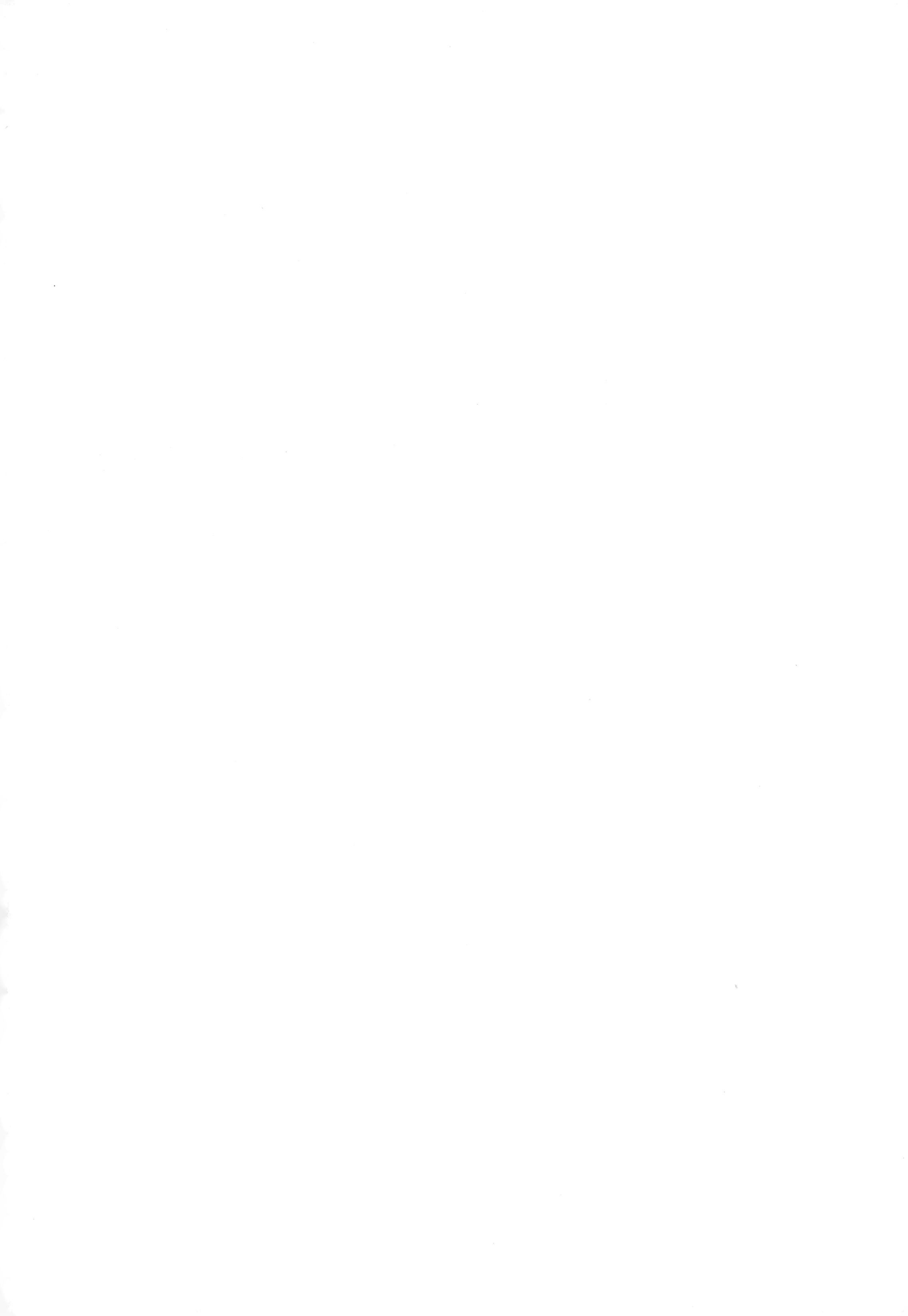

Chapter 7

Avoiding complications when using NobelGuide

Peter K Moy, Patrick Palacci, Ingvar Ericsson

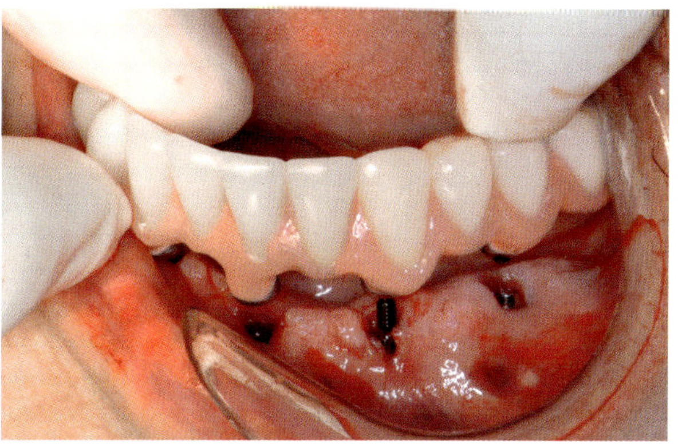

Difficulties and complications encountered with the NobelGuide technique may be considered according to three stages of treatment: during the workup and planning phase, the surgical procedure or the prosthodontic procedure.

As with any technique, the key to avoiding complications is anticipating where these problems may arise and taking the appropriate steps and measures to prevent their occurrence. The recommendations and solutions provided here are just some of the several methods for resolving potential problems, it is not intended to provide the reader with all of the solutions. However, with care and close attention to detail, many of the complications can be avoided, which is the best method for managing complications.

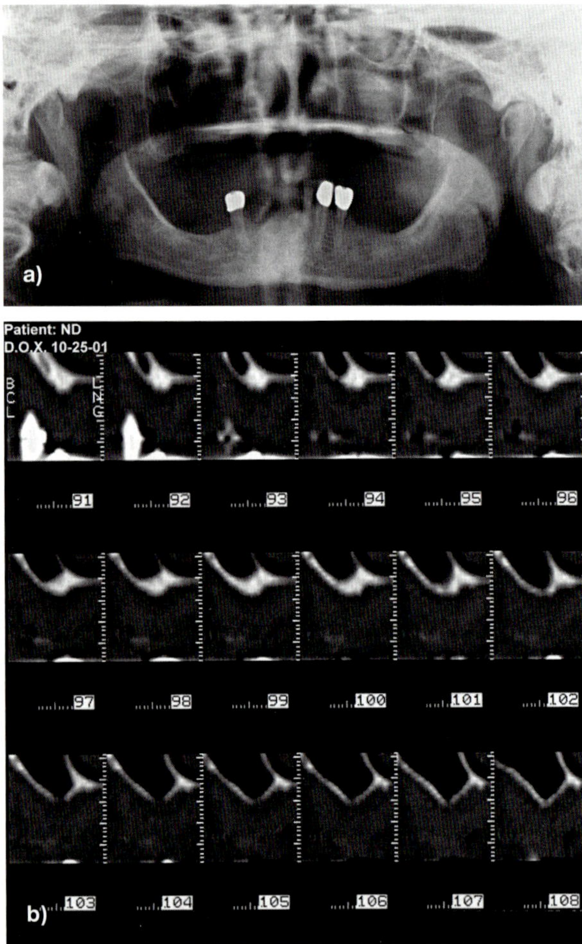

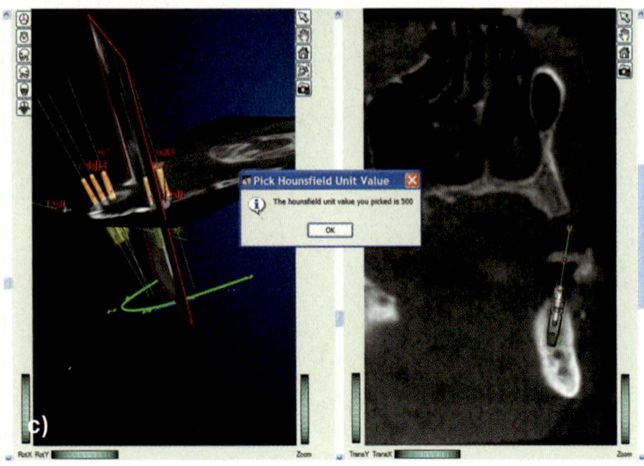

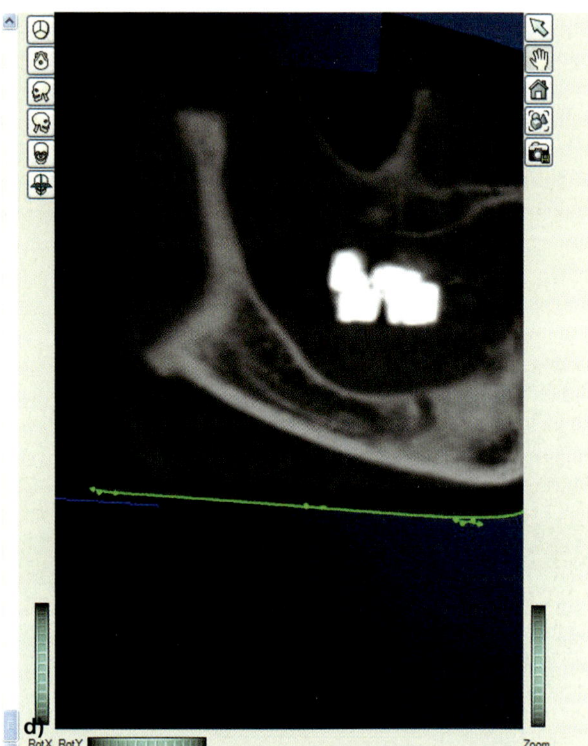

Fig 7-1 **(a)** Gross bone volume and available bone below the maxillary sinus cavity and above the inferior alveolar nerve. Accuracy is compromised by the variable magnification throughout the radiograph. **(b)** Computerized tomography (CT) scans of the maxillary sinus cavity are obtained to rule out disease pre-grafting or to determine the status of the maxillary sinus post-grafting. **(c)** Procera software reconstruction of the CT to assist in identifying the mandibular nerve canal. Software also enables viewing of three-dimensional (3D) planning (left screen) and measurement of bone density with Hounsfield units (right screen).
(d) Reconstruction of images in 3D permits identification of the inferior alveolar nerve canal and position of the mental foramina. As CT provides a 1:1 reproduction of the image size, accurate assessment of the available bone above the canal and foramina is possible.

Complications during planning

In guided surgery, pre-surgical planning may be performed using a model-based approach or computer software-based planning. Problems may be encountered using either method of planning.

Model-based planning

Inaccurate measurement of soft tissue thickness will result in improper representation of osseous ridge volume and/or contours. This will result in inaccurate positioning of the implant analog in the master model. This problem occurs with severe undercuts in the anterior maxilla or mandible, where access to measure gingival thickness is difficult.

It is inappropriate to use model-based planning for areas of the mouth that contain vital anatomic structures. Model-based planning is not indicated for the posterior quadrants of the intraoral cavity. The maxillary sinus and inferior alveolar nerve are vital structures that must be identified accurately on radiographs (Fig 7-1) and avoided in surgery. Accurate identification of these vital structures using model-based planning is not possible. Therefore, model-based planning should only be used for the anterior maxilla or mandible.

An inability to identify the position of adjacent root structures in relationship to the crest of the ridge is another reason to avoid using model-based planning. Even with appropriate radiographs, the convergence of adjacent roots makes model-based planning risky (Fig 7-2). The surgeon must be absolutely sure of where the root structures are positioned to avoid devitalizing the adjacent teeth.

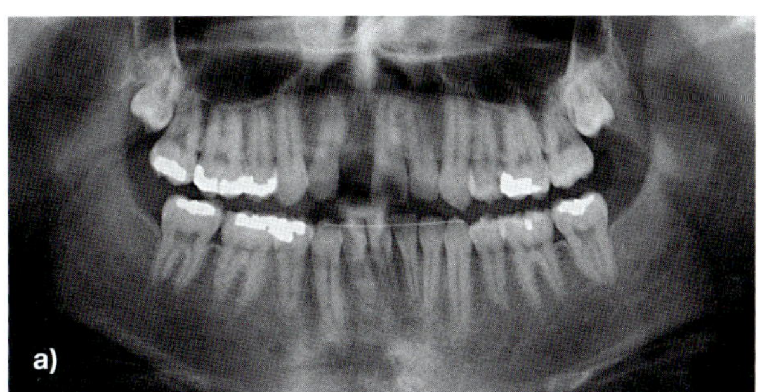

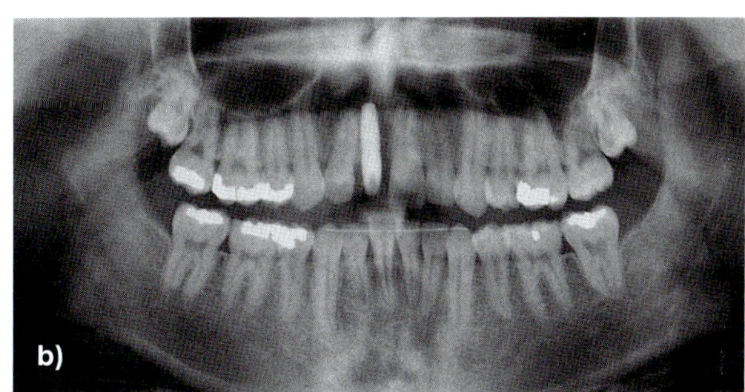

Fig 7-2 (a) A radiograph showing convergence of the roots of maxillary anterior teeth. Mesial–distal spacing between the roots of the right lateral incisor and left central incisor is very small. Model-based planning is contraindicated. **(b)** Identification of root positions with computerized tomography and use of a tapered-body implant assists in avoiding root structures and vital anatomy, such as the incisive foramen and canal.

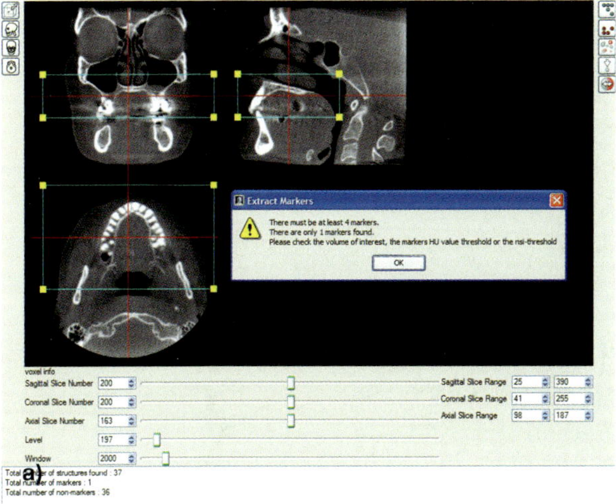

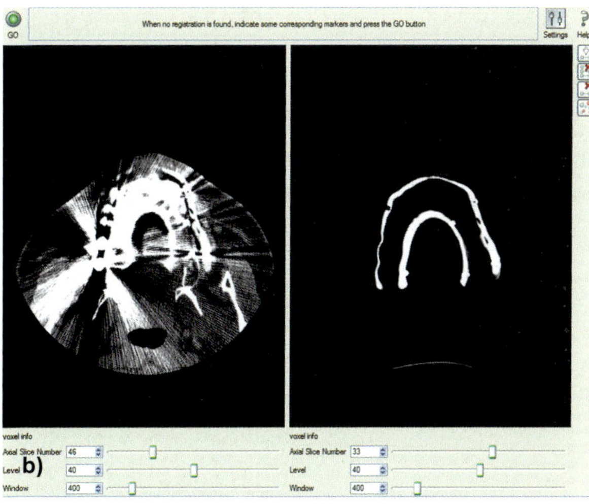

Fig 7-3 (a and b) Procera software must identify a minimum of four radiopaque markers on the scans of the patient and radiographic guide to superimpose the markers accurately and to allow superimposition of the prosthesis to the patient's bony anatomy.

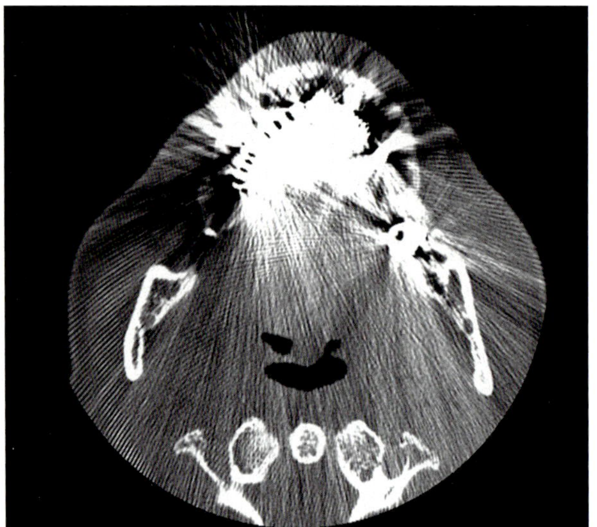

Fig 7-4 Scatter from the restorations covered radiopaque markers. It was not possible for the software to superimpose images of the markers and have an accurate correlation of the prosthesis to the patient's scan.

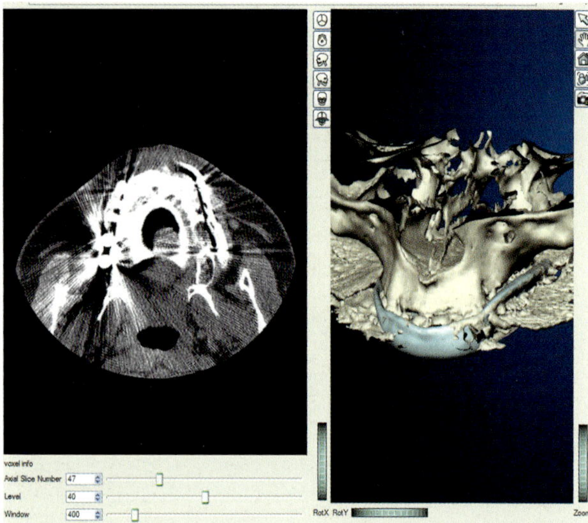

Fig 7-5 Owing to scatter from the metal restorations and the radiopaque guide, the contours of the alveolar ridge and dental structures are not visible.

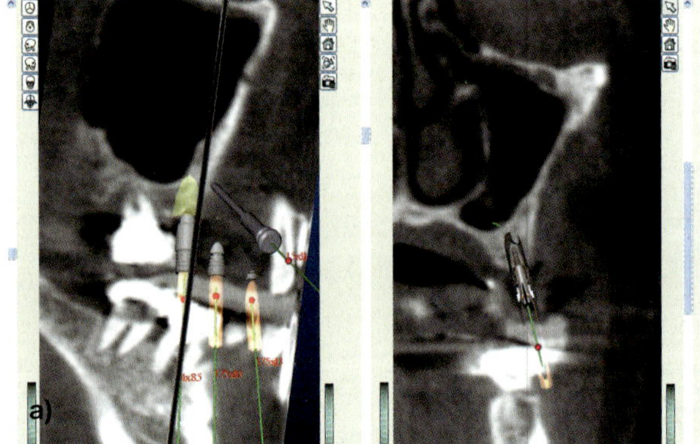

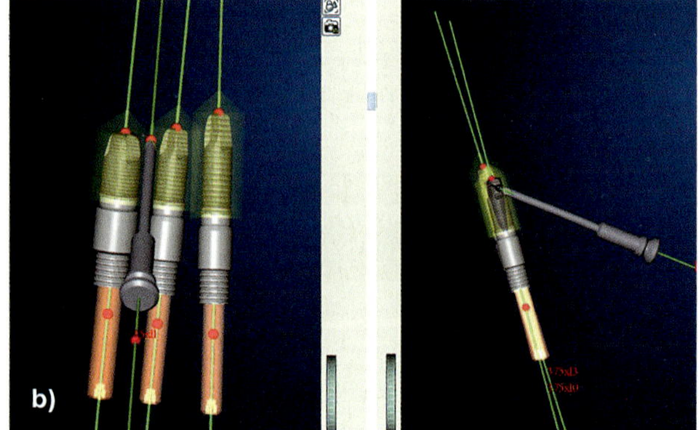

Fig 7-6 **(a)** A 'yellow zone' on the left screen indicates that the body of the implant is within 1.5 mm of the buccal surface of the alveolar ridge. **(b)** Superimposition of the yellow zone between implant bodies indicates there is 1.5 mm or less of bone between the two implants.

Computer-based planning

The inability to convert DICOM files with the original Procera software program occurred because it was not possible to superimpose or match up the radiopaque markers on the two scans: the scan of the patient and the scan of the radiographic guide (Fig 7-3). Markers may be hard to identify owing to scatter from adjacent metallic restorations, gutta-percha filling material in tooth roots superimposed on the markers, or the patient not wearing the radiographic guide during the scan (Fig 7-4). The newer version of the software program (Procera Software 2.0) permits conversion of the DICOM files of the patient scans without matching the radiopaque markers in the radiographic guide to the scans of the patient. However, if a radiographic guide is not used, visualization of a prosthesis superimposed over the patient scans will not be possible, thus the planning for implant positions will be less accurate.

The radiographic guide, when not properly designed or fabricated, may produce scatter owing to the use of certain soft re-line materials in the denture when attempting to obtain a more accurate intaglio surface. The re-line material may contain radiodense material, creating the scatter effect. When this occurs, the accuracy of the scan will be

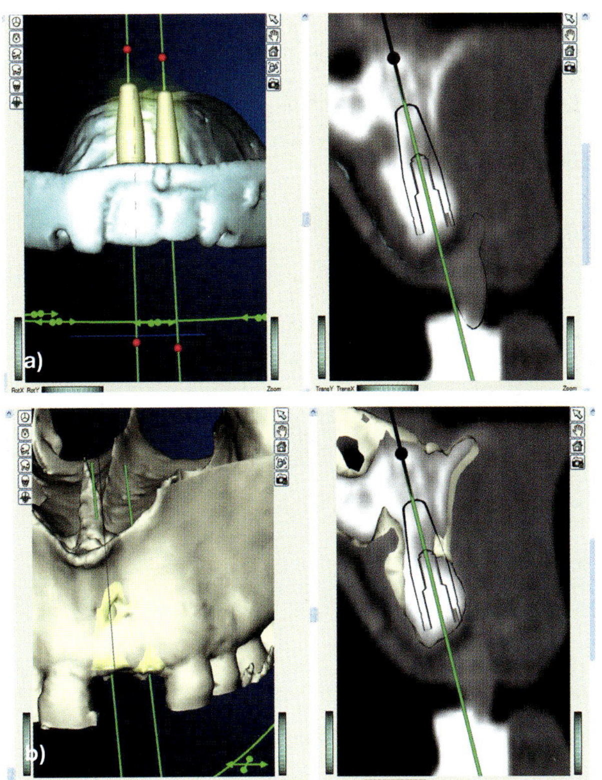

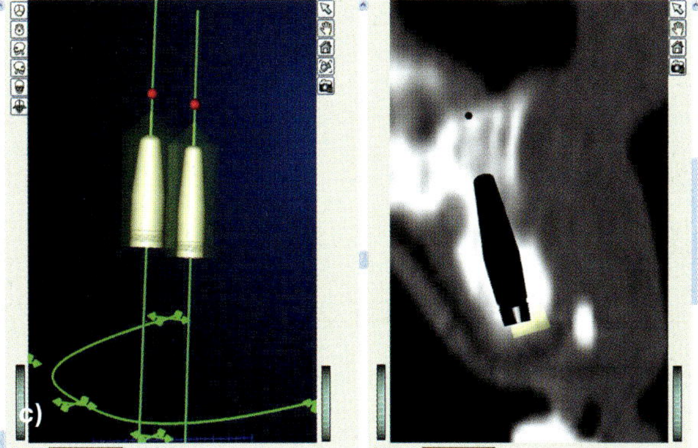

Fig 7-7 **(a)** Using tapered-body implants leaves more bone mass between the two implants at the apical one-third (left screen) and, more importantly, leaves more bone volume at the cortical aspects of the horizontally deficient alveolar ridge (right screen). **(b)** Even with a tapered body implant, the concavity at the subnasal region brings the body of the implant within 1.5 mm of the labial cortical bone. **(c)** Tapered body implant permits placement of the implant in a narrow ridge created by the incisive canal and the subnasal concavity.

reduced and the contours of the osseous structures difficult to visualize (Fig 7-5).

Problems may also be encountered through encroachment of the 'safety zone' (Fig 7-6), which is highlighted in yellow in the figure. This zone is a 1.5 mm wide area surrounding the implant body or other guided components on the software program. The safety zone surrounding the implant allows the clinician to be certain that the volume of bone between implants, or between the implant and buccal-lingual cortices of the alveolar, is sufficient to permit biologic osseointegration. The clinician performing the planning must remember the importance of a minimum of 1 mm width of bone laterally to cover the implant threads and 3 mm of bone between implants for adequate integration.

The safety zone surrounding other guided components will assure there is adequate space to permit the retention and stabilization of these components accurately within the surgical template. The safety zone will also permit the inspection of implant positions in three-dimensions (3D) so that the surgeon will be comfortable in placing the implants using flapless surgery (Fig 7-7).

The placement of the implant and/or components too deep or too superficial into the alveolar ridge during planning will generate an inaccurate surgical template. If the components are placed too far apically into the alveolar ridge, components may impinge on the osseous or gingival tissue, thus preventing the complete and accurate seating of the template (Fig 7-8). If the surgical template is not completely seated at the proper vertical dimension of occlusion or is seated with excessive compressive force on the mucosa, then all of the implants will be positioned too apically, with a final vertical dimension of occlusion that is open. Conversely, if the implants are not seated completely to the proper depth owing to improper assessment of the bone volume, and the compressive force on the mucosal tissue is inadequate, then the vertical positions of implants will be more superficial, resulting in prematurities or hyperocclusion from the prosthetic restoration being too high.

The final problem that may be encountered with

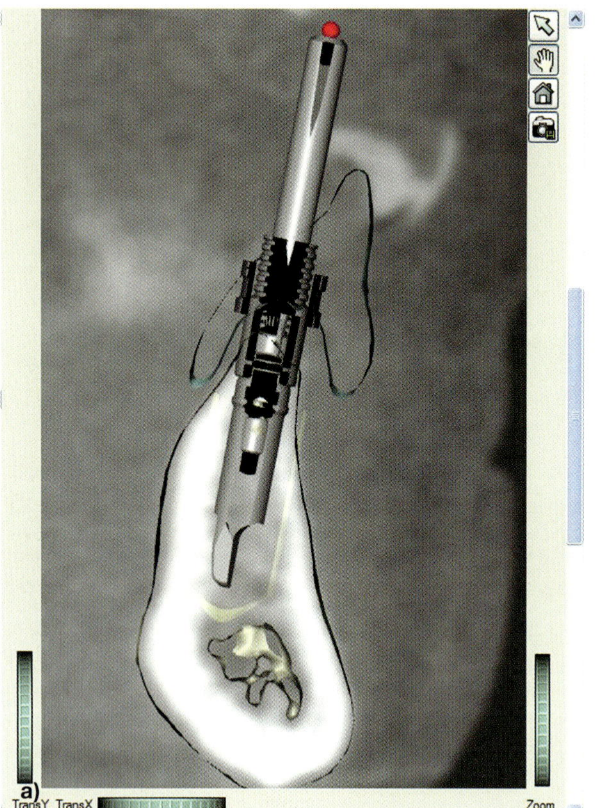

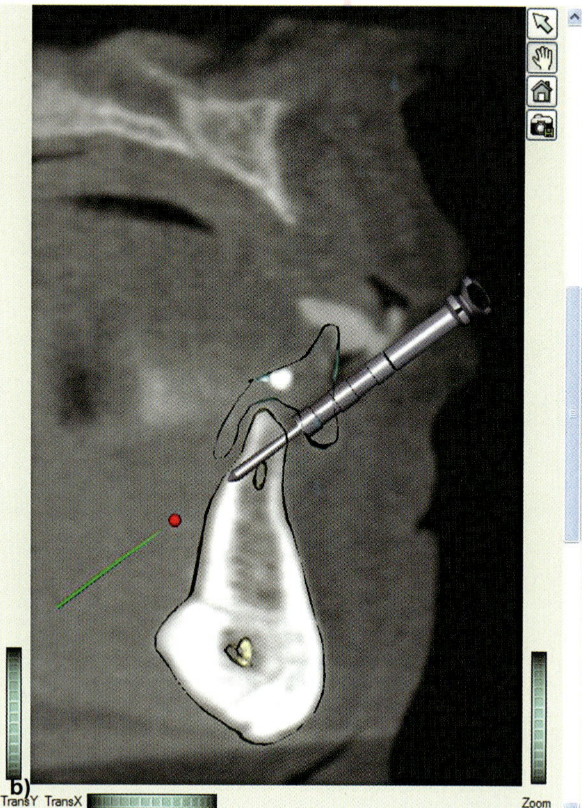

Fig 7-8 **(a)** Example of the guide cylinder placed too far inferiorly, which would impinge on the gingival tissue. Inferior margins of the guide cylinder are outside the confines of intaglio surface of the radiographic guide, which will result in the same position of the guide cylinder in the surgical template. This over-extended position of the cylinder would prohibit complete and accurate seating of the template. **(b)** A similar situation can occur with the guide cylinder used for the placement of horizontal anchor pins. Guide cylinders must be placed within the confines of the acrylic frame of the radiographic guide.

computer-based planning is failure to inspect the completed plan from a 3D perspective using features of the software program. This special feature permits inspection of the implant positions, as well as positions of all surgical components. Performing this inspection in 3D is an absolute requirement. Using two dimensions on the scans during implant positioning does not permit evaluation of proximity of components, especially at the apical regions of the implants. The separation of implants at the coronal aspect is guided by the pontics on the radiographic guide and easily visualized. However, the relative positions of the apical part of the implants are determined by mesial/distal and buccal-palatal/ lingual inclinations of the implant. Even though the coronal aspects of the implants may have adequate separation, the apical portion may be contacting owing to converging angulations of adjacent implants (Fig 7-9).

Complications during surgical procedure

Surgical access in the posterior quadrants, especially in the mandible, may be difficult when treating patients with limited opening. Owing to the additional thickness of the surgical template and constant length of the guide sleeves (10 mm), all drills are 10 mm longer. This requires the patient to be able to open 42 mm or more inter-incisally to permit access when surgery is performed in the posterior regions of the mouth (Fig 7-10).

Improper seating of the surgical template will result in the improper positioning of all implants, as well as affecting the occlusion provided by the prosthesis. It is imperative that the surgeon inserts the surgical template in the proper 3D position and vertical dimension of occlusion (Fig 7-11).

Incomplete seating of drills and implant mounts

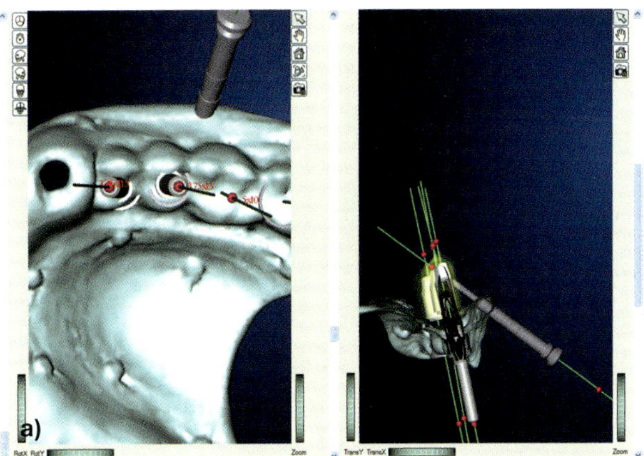

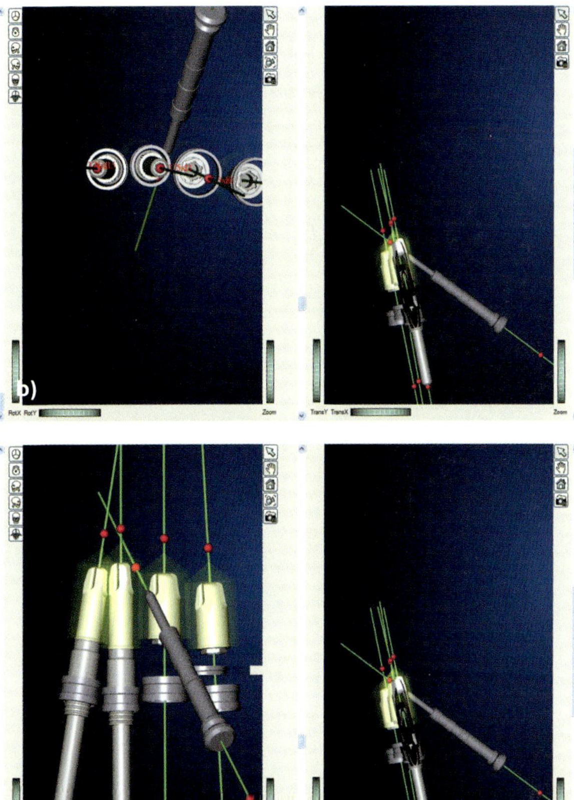

Fig 7-9 **(a)** The surgical template indicates adequate separation of the implant positions and cylinders at the occlusal surface. **(b)** Removing the outline of the surgical template, occlusal aspects of the guide cylinders appear to have adequate spacing between the cylinders. **(c)** Opposite view of the same workup, showing that apical aspects of the implants are in contact. This highlights the need for reviewing, at planning stage, the entire implant positions in three-dimensions, with the bone and radiographic guides removed.

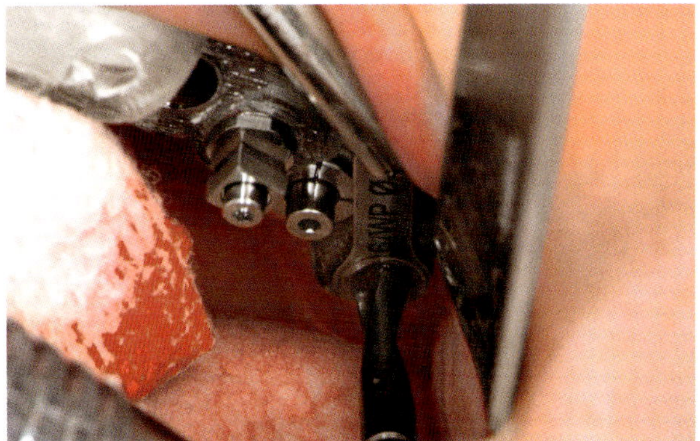

Fig 7-10 Use of extended drills and other components makes it extremely difficult to prepare molar sites.

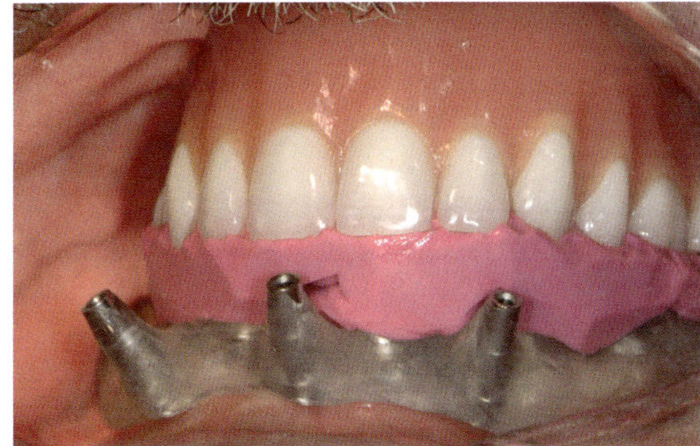

Fig 7-11 Insertion of the surgical template must be accurate in three-dimensions, especially in re-establishing the proper vertical dimension of occlusion. Note the surgical index, which aligns the surgical template with the opposing dentition or prosthesis.

on to the guide sleeves will result in underpreparation of the implant site and leads to incomplete vertical seating of the implant (Fig 7-12), leaving the head of the implant super-crestal or outside of the alveolar ridge contours. This will place the prosthesis in the improper vertical plane and in hyperocclusion.

When alveolar ridges in either jaw are significantly resorbed, it will be difficult to retain the surgical template and maintain an accurate position during the surgical procedure (Figs 7-13 and 7-14). There are also vital structures on the lingual aspect of the mandibular ridge, as well as the floor of the nose and maxillary sinuses that may be at greater risk for injury (Fig 7-14).

Flapless procedures do not permit visualization of the surgical sites, thus making it difficult to correct

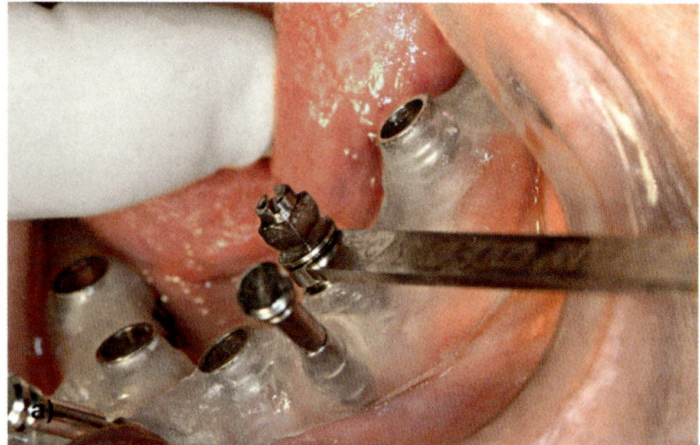

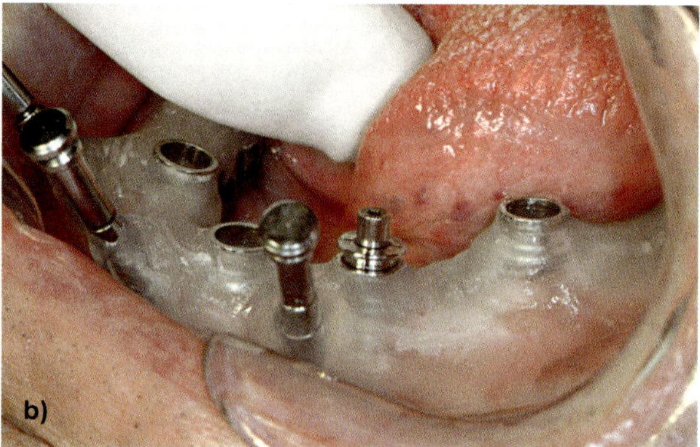

Fig 7-12 **(a)** The fixture mount (implant carrier) is not completely seated, indicating that the site was not prepared properly or the implant is not completely seated. **(b)** As the implant was not completely seated, all other components that are attached to the implant will have the same discrepancy. The template abutment is not in contact with the surgical template's guide cylinder.

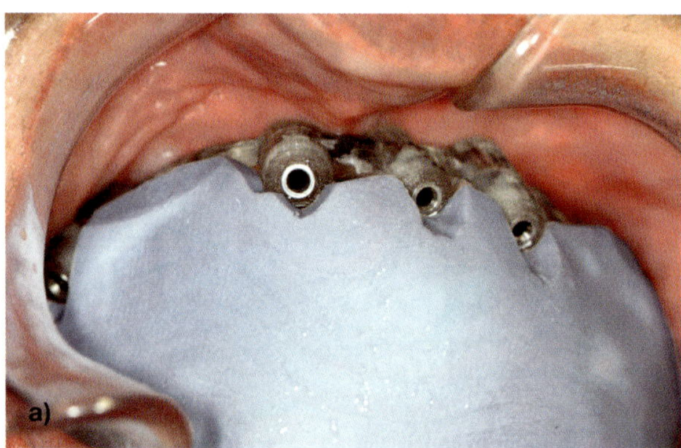

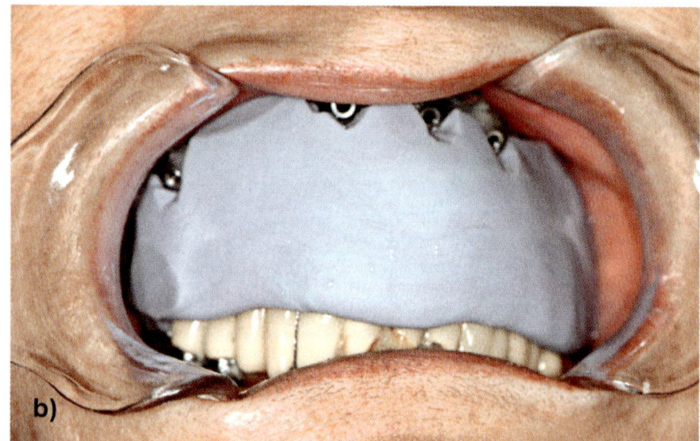

Fig 7-13 **(a)** A severely resorbed maxillary arch. Note the thickness of the surgical index, which may have inherent inaccuracies with the seating of the surgical template. **(b)** Full view of the vertical dimension and establishment of the template position by indexing to the opposing occlusion.

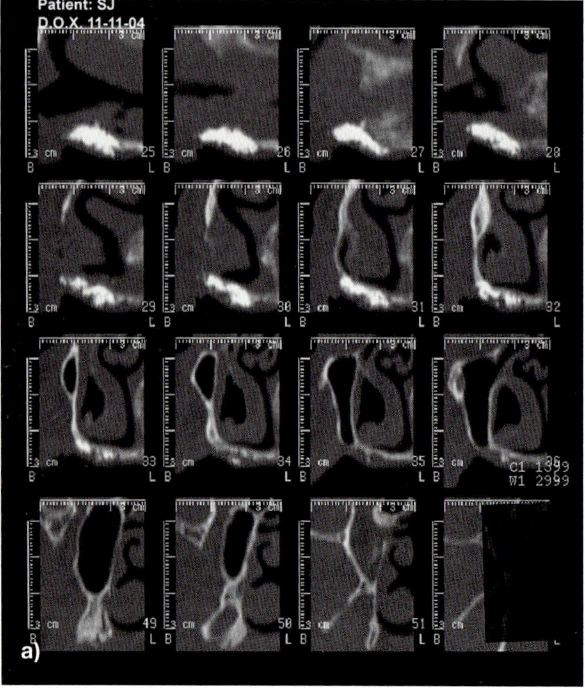

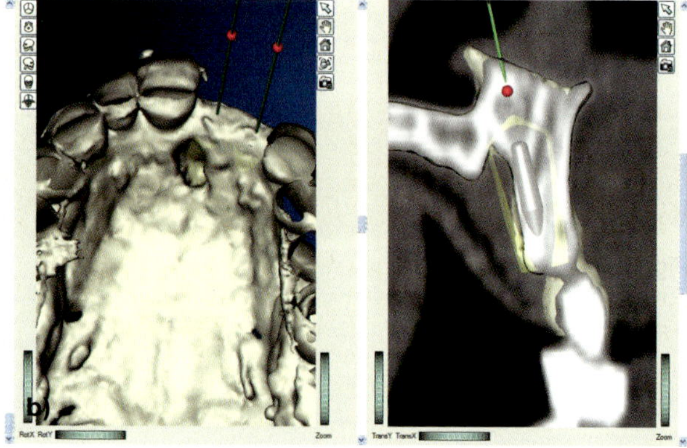

Fig 7-14 **(a)** A maxillary computerized tomographic scan showing severe resorption of the maxilla, extending from anterior (showing the incisive canal) to posterior (showing resorption of the alveolar ridge below the sinus cavity and the tuberosity/pterygoid plates). **(b)** Occlusal view of the maxilla, showing the large incisive foramina extending into the alveolar ridge.

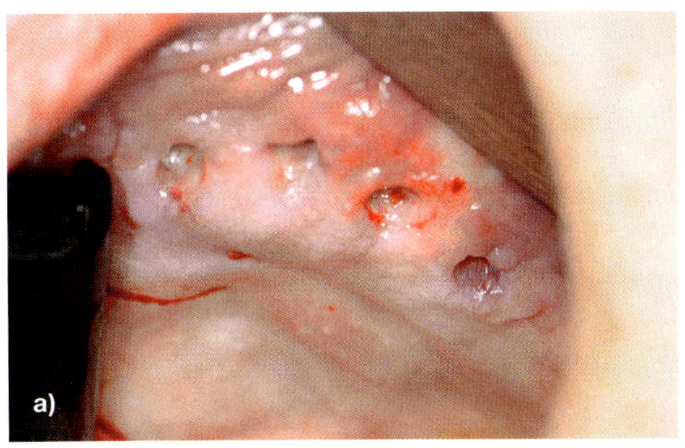
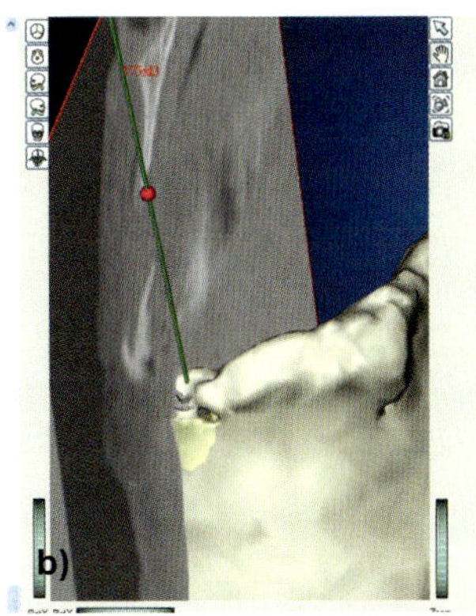
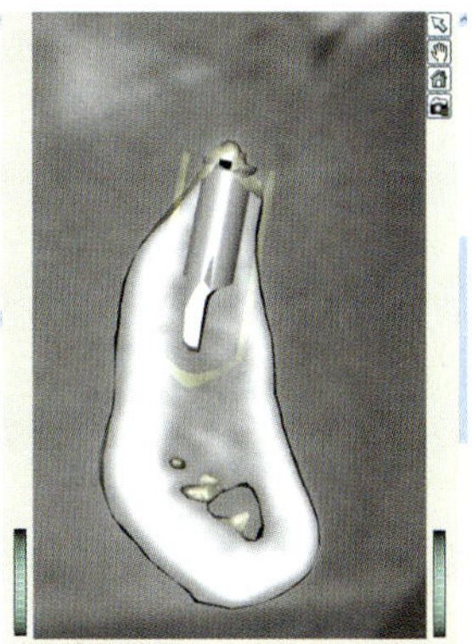

Fig 7-15 **(a)** Flapless surgical approach does not permit viewing of alveolar ridge irregularities or impingement of soft tissue. **(b)** Severely resorbed, knife-edge ridge will typically have a higher lingual or palatal cortical plate of bone. This ledge of bone often impedes complete seating of the prosthesis.

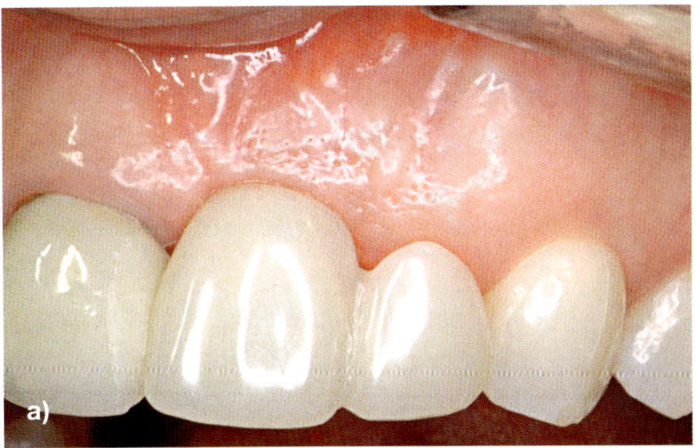
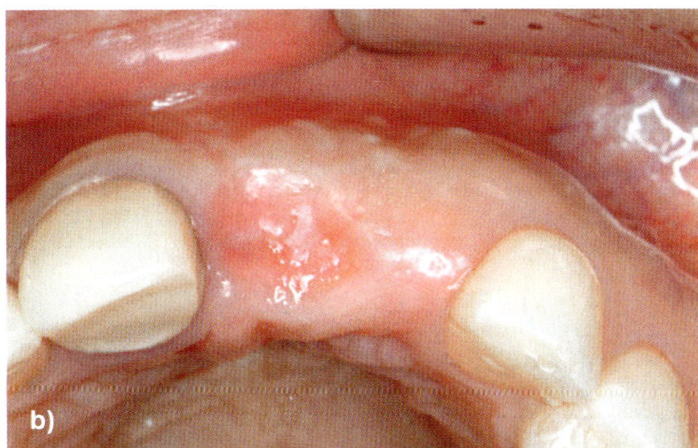
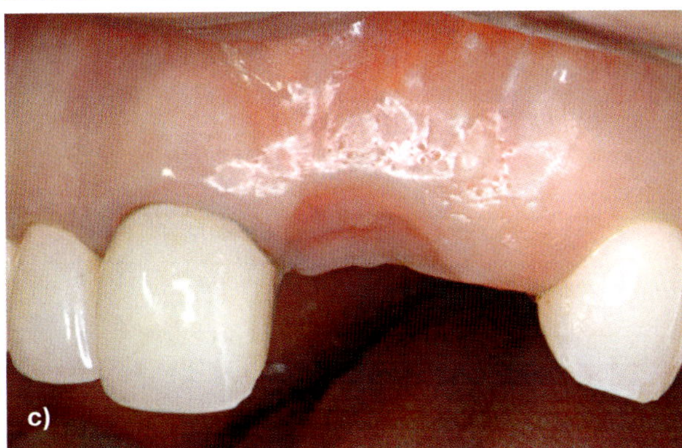
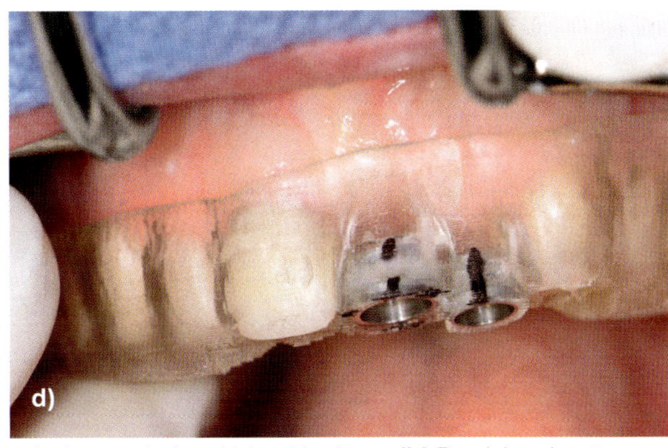

Fig 7-16 **(a)** Preoperative view of provisional prosthesis replacing missing central and lateral incisors. **(b)** Provisional restoration removed to show the edentulous ridge contour and soft tissue volume. **(c)** Occlusal view showing adequate width and gingival biotype. **(d)** Partially dentate surgical template for minimally invasive surgery.

anatomic deficiencies of the alveolar ridge (Fig 7-15). These deficiencies may inhibit complete seating of the prosthesis, especially in the anterior ridge where knife-edged ridges are often encountered. After preparing the osseous site, the thin lingual or palatal cortical ridge remains, which will impede the complete seating of the prosthetic or guided abutments.

Placement of implants too close to each other or using abutments that are too wide in diameter will result in loss of interproximal papilla (Fig 7-16). This is especially crucial to avoid in the esthetic zone.

When natural teeth are adjacent to an edentulous site, the surgical template may be too thin and have insufficient bulk of acrylic to secure the guide cylinders that direct the drills and implant placement (Fig 7-17). These areas of the surgical teme)

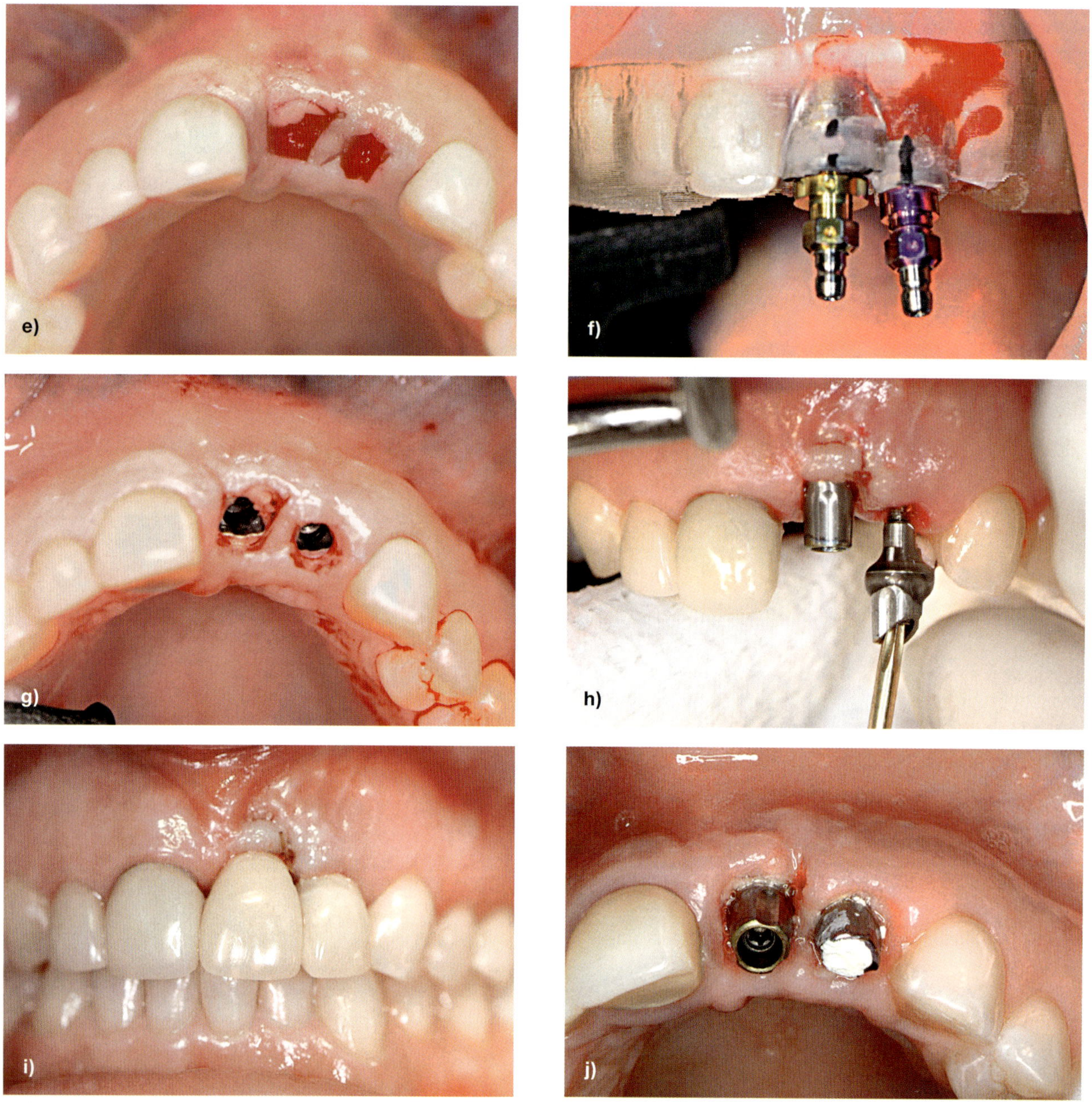

f)

g)

h)

i)

j)

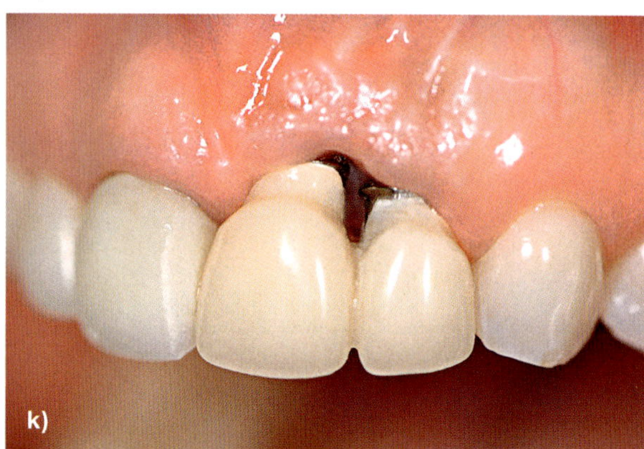

Fig 7-16 **(e)** Central incisor region with a small flap to maintain tissue volume on the labial aspect. In the lateral incisor area a tissue punch was used. **(f)** Implants were inserted using a guided surgical technique. **(g)** Occlusal view with implants in final position. **(h)** Delivery of definitive abutments. Note the wide circumferential dimensions of the abutment that is subgingival, especially for a lateral incisor. **(i)** Delivery of the provisional restorations. **(j)** Occlusal view of the prosthetic abutments and limited spacing interproximally. **(k)** Two-week status after minimally invasive surgery and immediate function. Gingival tissue has receded, owing to tight inter-implant spacing and loss of blood supply to this area.

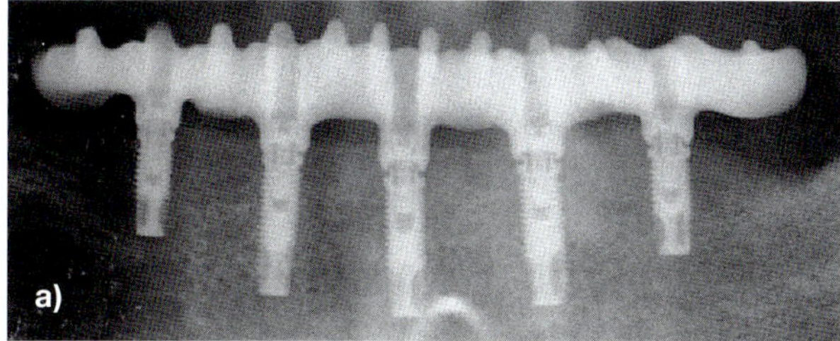

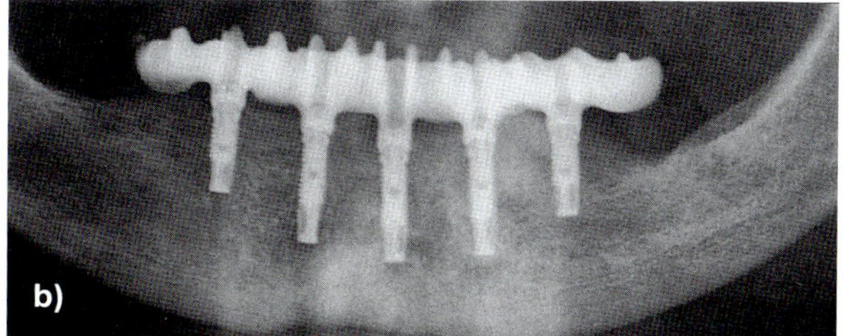

Fig 7-17 **(a)** Panoramic radiograph after delivery of prosthesis, showing incomplete seating of the framework because of the knife-edge ridge found in the anterior mandible. **(b)** After using a bone mill to clear off excess bone, the prosthetic frame was completely seated.

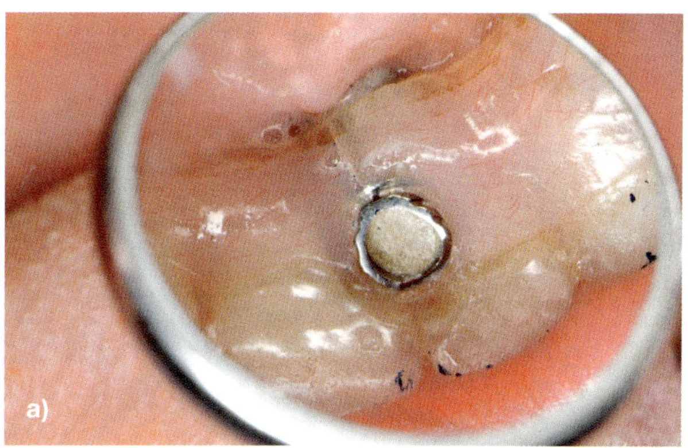

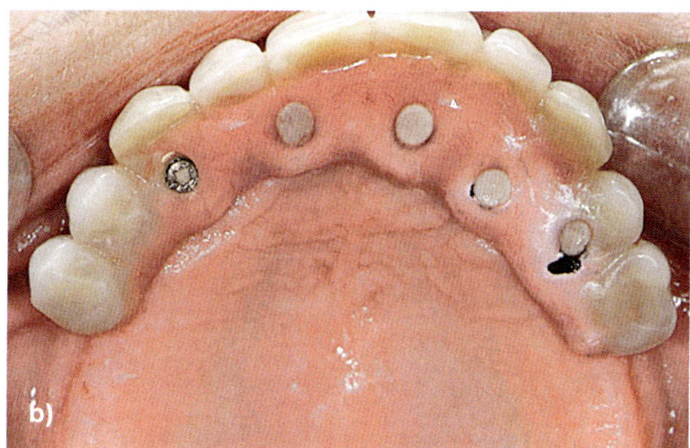

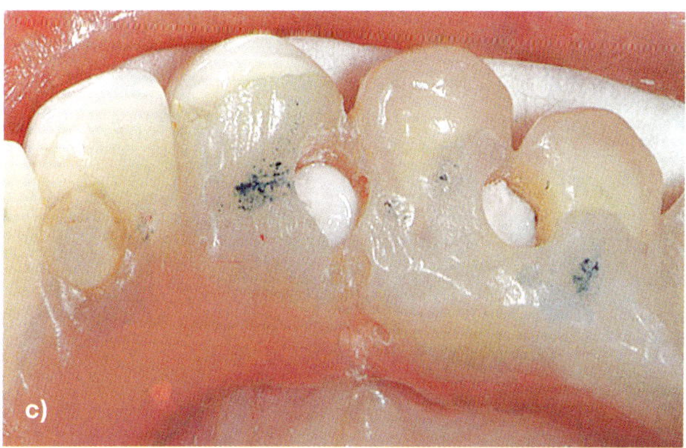

Fig 7-18 (a–c) Fracture lines in the acrylic frame extending through the access sleeve.

plate are prone to fracturing or splintering under the pressures applied to the template during the surgical procedure.

Complications during prosthodontic procedure

Loosening of guided abutment screws leads to a loose prosthesis. This complication occurred with a higher frequency when the prosthetic framework was made with reinforced carbon fiber acrylic (Fig 7-18).

Incomplete seating of the prosthetic bridge results in malocclusion. This may occur when the bone from the thin alveolar ridge is not completely removed. If this bone remains, it will impede full seating of the guided abutments (Fig 7-19).

Problems may be encountered with fracturing of acrylic veneers or denture teeth, which also occur with higher frequency when the all-acrylic framework is used (Fig 7-20).

Finally, gingival hyperplasia and mucosal reactions have been associated with poor oral hygiene (Fig 7-21). This is especially true with a full fixed prosthesis that overlaps the edentulous ridge, making it difficult for patient to access with hygiene instruments. Therefore, it is important to ensure that the patient is aware of the need and importance of oral hygiene before commencing with the prosthodontic procedure.

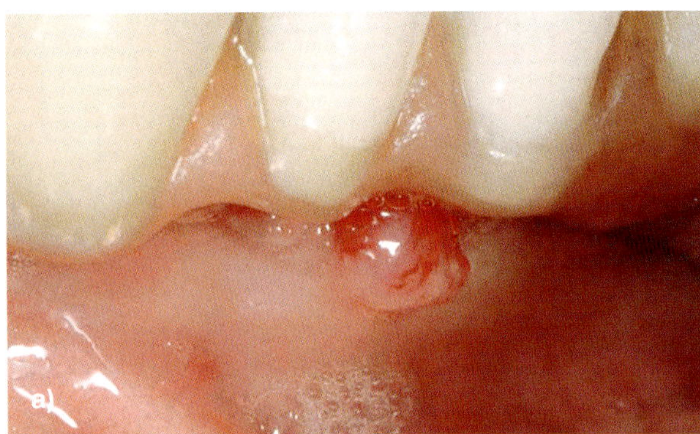

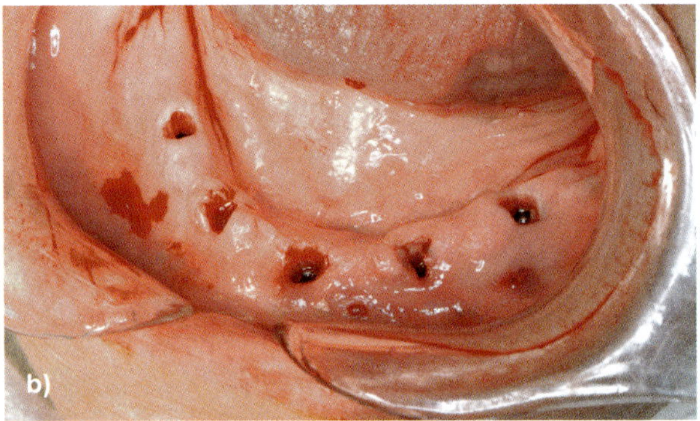

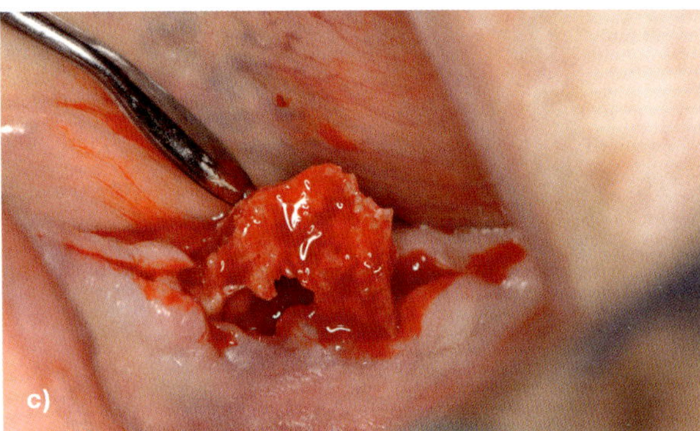

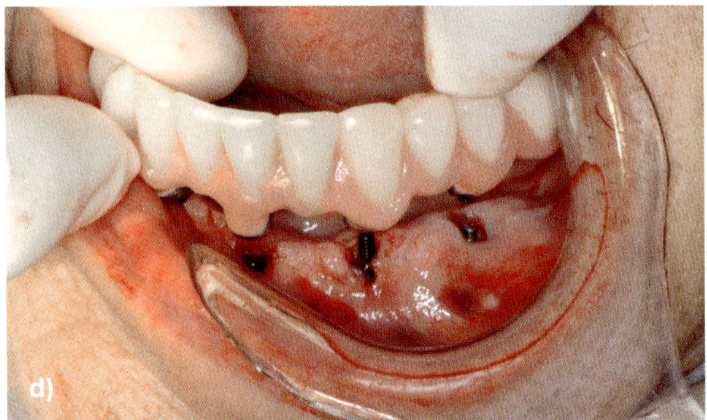

Fig 7-19 **(a)** Flapless surgery does not permit easy access to excess bone typically found on the thin lingual ridge. **(b)** Creating a small flap to expose the excess bone will permit easy removal and alleviate the impingement. **(c and d)** The prosthetic frame is now easily delivered into position.

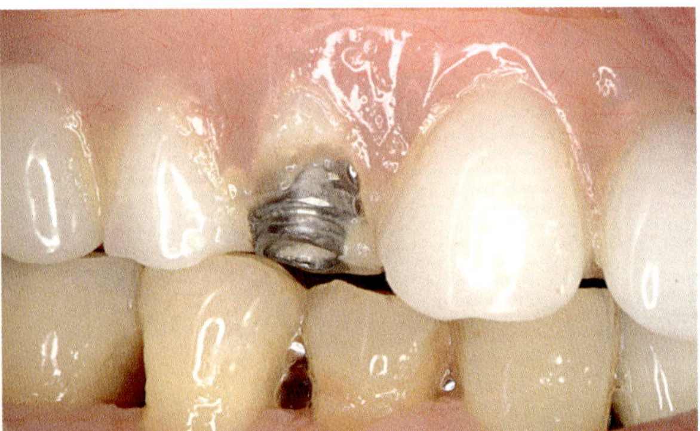

Fig 7-20 Delaminating of pontic denture tooth from the acrylic frame of the prosthesis.

Conclusion

The examples given illustrate that there are relatively few complications associated with the NobelGuide technique, as long as the clinician performs the guided procedures correctly, and that such complications are easily avoided or managed through proper assessment of the CT scans and appropriate planning with the Procera software program. The clinician should be aware that many of the complications highlighted may be preventable by taking appropriate precautions and care during all phases of treatment for immediate function and loading of implants.

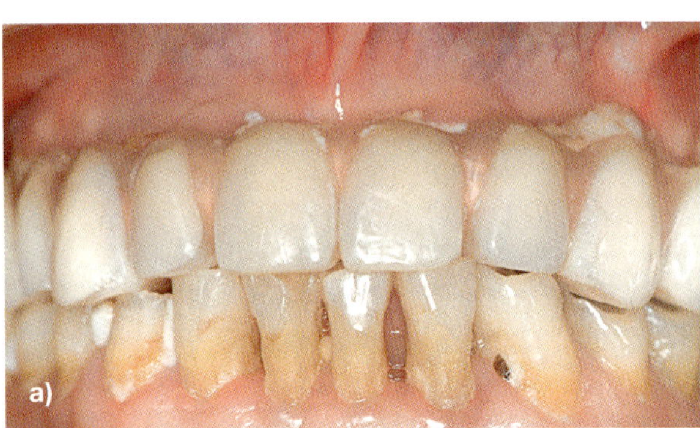

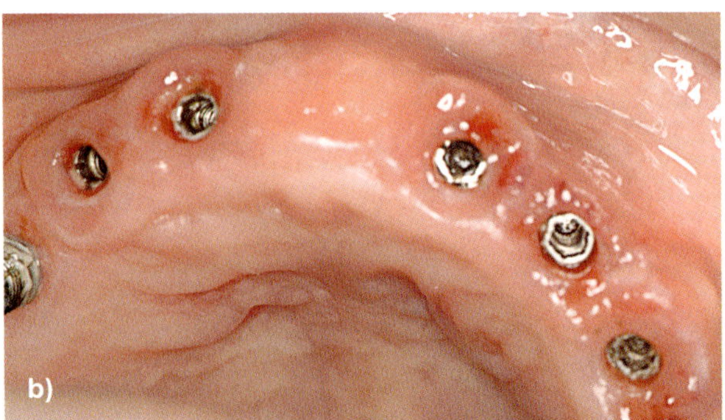

Fig 7-21 **(a)** Poor oral hygiene will lead to inflammatory reactions and gingival hyperplasia. **(b)** Fixed prosthesis has been removed and inflamed mucosa is visible, especially surrounding the neck of the implants. If this persists, the inflammatory reaction will lead to bone loss.

Chapter 8

Conclusion

Peter K Moy, Patrick Palacci, Ingvar Ericsson

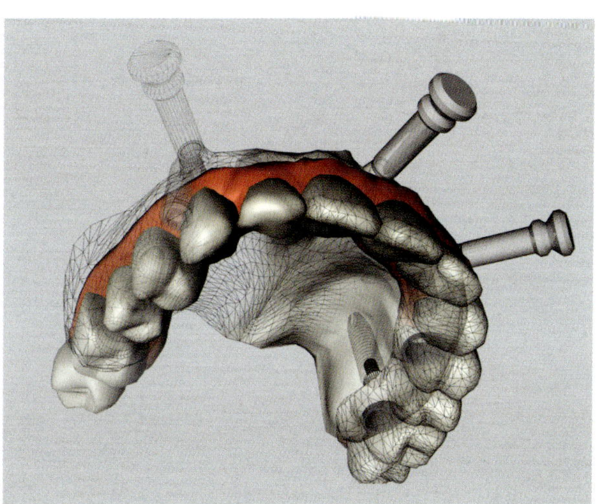

For decades, practitioners have successfully placed implants with limited diagnostic tools for the workup and planning. The technology previously available included flat film radiology, such as peri-apical, panoramic or lateral cephalometric radiographs. More recently, computerized tomographic (CT) images taken by medical scanners are reconstructed using computer software programs to reformat the scanned images and provide a more accurate, three-dimensional image. Even with these advanced radiographic analyses, the proper placement and ultimate position of implants were dependent on the clinician's ability and level of experience.

However, with the development and refinement of modern computer software programs, this digital information permits a more comprehensive understanding and knowledge of the patient's bone anatomy, location of critical vital structures, such as the inferior alveolar nerve, and hard and soft tissue defects. With advanced knowledge of the location of critical anatomical landmarks, the clinician can avoid these deficient sites and vital structures and, more importantly, recommend corrective surgical procedures to augment and correct the deficiencies.

The success and predictability of dental implant treatment has and will continue to progress. Diagnostic tools will continue to improve and it is anticipated the improvements will provide the clinician with the ability to determine bone volume and density with a precision that will make the goal of achieving 99% success with implants that are immediately loaded a distinct possibility.

Improvements in this area also allow the clinician to optimize implant positioning in harmony with future prosthetic restoration by using specially designed surgical templates generated with information obtained from CT for guided implant placement: the primary goal of the NobelGuide concept. This optimal positioning of implants will provide a better soft tissue environment by respecting the interproximal spacing between implants or between the implant and tooth.

Optimizing inter-implant or implant–tooth spacing maintains adequate blood supply, avoids overcompression of peri-implant soft tissue with the contours of the implant abutment or restoration and allows access for proper oral hygiene maintenance. Regardless of the many benefits that a guided surgical concept affords the clinician, the experience and skills of the clinician remain vitally important to achieving a successful treatment outcome. Surgical judgment and proper intra- and postoperative management are essential for avoiding complications and negative outcomes. When faced with an intraoperative complication, the clinician must rely on past experience with open-flap techniques to manage many of the problems that may arise from minimally invasive or flapless procedures. Modern technology and concepts can assist in improving success and predictability with dental implant therapy, but they cannot replace the surgical and prosthodonthic skills and acumen required of the clinician.

The concept of NobelGuide is to provide information that permits fabrication of the prosthetic restoration prior to the surgical procedure. This is possible through the generation of a surgical template that will guide the surgeon in the placement of dental implants into desired, pre-planned positions, as dictated by the definitive prosthesis. The technology and procedural steps associated with NobelGuide can be used for several purposes:

- guiding implant placement following the demands and requirements of the definitive restoration
- diagnosis by measuring bone density and determining the need for performing grafting or augmentation procedures with site specificity, prior to or simultaneously with implant placement
- providing a surgical tool (surgical template) to assist in implant placement for basic and advanced surgical cases, as well as for minimally invasive flapless surgery for all clinical states of edentulism
- indicating to the laboratory technician the exact location of the final implant positions so that the framework and the prosthesis may be fabricated prior to the actual surgical procedure
- co-ordinating surgical and prosthodontic treatments to include placement of a provisional or definitive restoration immediately after implant placement.

The range of clinical applications that is currently being developed will certainly increase in the future as the evolution of computer software programs, surgical instrumentation, dental materials and technology continues to improve. The future for the clinician to provide immediate function and immediate esthetics for patients requiring dental implants is extremely promising.

Index

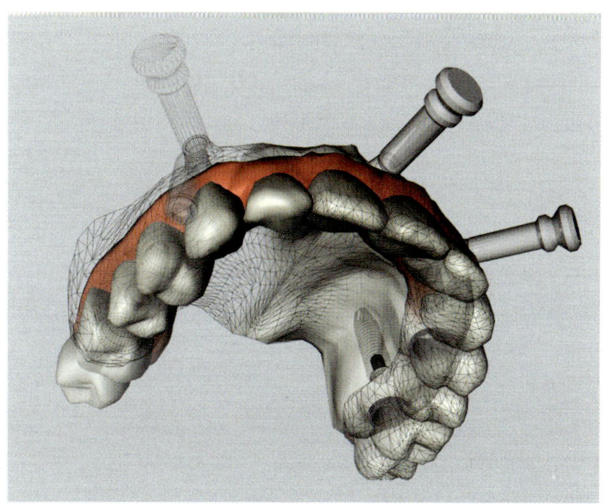

A

B

C

D

E

F

G

H

I

R

S

T

V

W

Z